ANGER MANAGEMENT FOR EXPLOSIVE PARENTS

Be The Master Of Your Emotions

Megan G. Mansfield

Table of contents

8.2.2 Staying Committed to Personal Growth

Conclusion

Introduction

In the chaotic tapestry of parenthood, where the threads of joy and challenges intricately weave together, we extend a heartfelt welcome to a transformative expedition. This literary voyage, encapsulated in "Anger Management for Explosive Parents: Be the Master of Your Emotions," invites you to embark on a profound odyssey of self-discovery, emotional intelligence, and ultimately, the cultivation of harmonious familial connections.

At the core of this endeavor lies a distinct purpose — to provide a compass for parents grappling with explosive anger, offering not just theoretical insights but tangible tools that pave the way toward emotional mastery. The intention is clear: to facilitate an exploration of emotions, empowering parents with the skills to navigate the turbulent seas of anger, fostering an environment wherein both parent and child can flourish emotionally and relationally.

To comprehend the depths of explosive anger in parents, we embark on a journey of introspection. What triggers these intense emotional reactions, and what intricate emotional patterns contribute to these tumultuous outbursts? Our exploration is guided by compassion, seeking to unravel the intricacies of these emotional currents. Through this understanding, we empower parents to address the root causes, providing a solid foundation for transformative change.

The roots of explosive anger often stretch deep into our personal histories, shaped by experiences that have left an indelible mark on our emotional landscapes. As we navigate this terrain, we will examine the impact of childhood influences and societal expectations, acknowledging that the journey toward emotional mastery involves untangling complex webs woven over years.

Anger, a natural and potent emotion, takes center stage in our exploration. Unbridled, it can transform from a fleeting emotional response into a disruptive force, particularly within the intimate confines of a family. Understanding the profound importance of anger management becomes our lodestar. This book is dedicated to equipping you with the knowledge and practical tools necessary to skillfully navigate the labyrinth of emotions, fostering a home environment characterized by understanding, empathy, and love.

The significance of this journey lies not merely in the cessation of explosive anger but in the cultivation of emotional intelligence — an awareness and acceptance of one's own emotions and the ability to respond to them in a healthy and constructive manner. Through this process, we aspire to create a haven where familial bonds are fortified by open communication, mutual respect, and a shared journey of growth.

As we embark on this journey together, it is crucial to recognize that personal growth is not a sprint but a marathon, a continuous process of self-reflection and refinement. The insights, strategies, and exercises presented in the following chapters are not quick fixes but rather companions on a lifelong journey of emotional mastery.

The path to becoming the master of your emotions is characterized by self-compassion, resilience, and an unwavering commitment to personal growth. It is a path where every step, no matter how small, contributes to the creation of a home environment that transcends the challenges of explosive anger, embracing a culture of compassion, communication, and tranquility.

May this book be your guide, offering support and insights as you navigate the intricate terrain of your emotions. Let it serve as a beacon, guiding you toward a destination where you, as a parent, hold the reins of your emotional well-being, steering towards a home filled with understanding, love, and enduring serenity.

Chapter 1: The Impact of Explosive Parental Anger

1.1 Effects on Children

In the intricate dance of parent-child relationships, emotions play a pivotal role. The impact of a parent's emotional state, particularly when characterized by explosive anger, can be profound and lasting. In this chapter, we delve into the intricate web of effects on children, emphasizing the critical role that effective anger management plays in fostering a nurturing and emotionally healthy environment.

The Ripple Effect of Parental Anger

Children, like emotional sponges, absorb the energy and atmosphere around them. When parents grapple with explosive anger, the reverberations are felt keenly by their offspring. Emotional turmoil within the parental sphere often translates into a heightened sense of anxiety and insecurity for children. Their world, ideally a haven of love and support, becomes tinged with unpredictability and fear.

1. Emotional Impact: Explosive anger creates an emotional landscape that is both tumultuous and unpredictable. Children, who are still developing their emotional regulation skills, struggle to comprehend and navigate this terrain. The constant exposure to anger can lead to heightened stress levels, manifesting in emotional distress, anxiety, and even depression.

2. Behavioral Consequences: The behavioral manifestations of parental anger are diverse and impactful. Children may internalize the explosive behavior, leading to self-esteem issues or externalize it through defiant or aggressive behavior. Academic performance may suffer, as the emotional burden becomes a hindrance to cognitive development.

The Cycle of Generational Patterns

One cannot discuss the effects of parental anger without acknowledging the potential perpetuation of generational patterns. Children observe and learn from their parents, and without intervention, the cycle of explosive anger may persist from one generation to the next.

1. Modeling Behavior: Children often model their behavior based on what they observe at home. If explosive anger is the predominant mode of emotional expression, children may internalize this as an acceptable way to deal with frustration and stress, perpetuating the cycle in their own lives and future relationships.

2. Communication Patterns: Effective communication is a cornerstone of healthy relationships. Parental anger can disrupt these patterns, teaching children that aggression is a viable means of expressing oneself. This distorted communication

model may hinder their ability to form positive connections with others.

Long-Term Consequences

The impact of explosive parental anger extends beyond the immediate emotional and behavioral consequences, influencing the trajectory of a child's life well into adulthood.

1. Interpersonal Relationships: Children raised in an environment characterized by explosive anger may struggle with forming and maintaining healthy relationships. Trust issues, difficulty expressing emotions, and challenges in resolving conflicts amicably are common themes that persist into adulthood.

2. Emotional Regulation: The ability to regulate emotions is a crucial life skill. Children exposed to unmanaged anger may encounter difficulties in this area, potentially leading to mental health challenges such as

anxiety disorders and issues related to impulse control.

The Role of Anger Management in Parenting

Understanding the profound impact of explosive anger on children underscores the critical importance of effective anger management for parents. It's not merely about controlling emotions but creating a conducive emotional environment for the holistic development of the child.

1. Modeling Healthy Emotion Regulation: By mastering their own emotions, parents become powerful role models for their children. Demonstrating healthy anger management techniques teaches children constructive ways to navigate their own emotional landscapes.

2. Creating Emotional Safety: A home characterized by controlled and managed emotions fosters a sense of emotional safety

for children. Knowing that their parents can navigate challenges without explosive anger creates a stable and secure environment for emotional growth.

3. Promoting Effective Communication: Anger management is intrinsically linked to effective communication. Parents who master their emotions can engage in open, honest, and constructive dialogue with their children, laying the foundation for positive relationships and conflict resolution skills.

In navigating the effects of explosive parental anger on children, the path to emotional mastery becomes not only a personal journey but a legacy of resilience and emotional well-being passed down through generations. In the subsequent chapters, we will explore in-depth strategies for recognizing and managing triggers, understanding the roots of anger, and ultimately becoming the master of your emotions for the benefit of yourself and the ones you hold most dear—the next generation.

1.1.1 Emotional Impact

Navigating the intricate landscape of emotions within the realm of parenthood requires a keen understanding of the profound emotional impact explosive anger can have on both parents and their children. In this exploration, we delve into the multifaceted dimensions of the emotional impact, emphasizing the transformative potential of effective anger management. By becoming the master of one's emotions, parents not only reclaim control over their internal world but also foster an environment where emotional well-being can flourish.

The Tumultuous Seas of Parental Anger

Explosive anger, a tempestuous force within the familial dynamic, creates emotional ripples that extend far beyond the immediate moment of eruption. To comprehend its emotional impact, we must first acknowledge the sheer intensity and unpredictability that characterize such outbursts. Children, in particular, bear witness to this emotional turbulence, leaving an indelible mark on their own emotional landscapes.

1. Stress and Anxiety: Children, often unable to articulate the complexity of their emotions, internalize the stress and anxiety generated by explosive anger. The home, ideally a sanctuary of safety and comfort, transforms into a battleground of emotional uncertainty. The constant tension can manifest in a heightened state of vigilance, contributing to a pervasive sense of insecurity.

2. Emotional Distress: The emotional distress experienced by children in the aftermath of explosive anger is a poignant reality. Feelings of fear, sadness, and confusion become intertwined with their

daily experiences, shaping their emotional responses and influencing their perceptions of the world around them.

The Burden on Parental Well-being

While the focus often centers on the impact on children, it's crucial to recognize the toll explosive anger takes on parental well-being. Parents, grappling with the aftermath of emotional outbursts, may find themselves ensnared in a cycle of guilt, remorse, and heightened stress.

1. Guilt and Shame: The aftermath of explosive anger is often accompanied by a wave of guilt and shame. Parents, recognizing the impact on their children, may internalize these emotions, creating a pervasive sense of inadequacy. Breaking free from this cycle requires not only mastering anger but also cultivating self-compassion.

2. Strained Parent-Child Relationships: Explosive anger strains the delicate fabric of parent-child relationships. The emotional distance that ensues can hinder the development of a secure attachment, essential for a child's emotional and social well-being. Addressing this emotional chasm necessitates a commitment to self-awareness and transformative change.

The Transformative Power of Anger Management

Understanding the emotional impact of explosive anger serves as the impetus for transformative change. Anger management, when approached as a holistic endeavor, becomes a powerful tool for parents to reclaim control over their emotions and cultivate a nurturing environment for their children.

1. Cultivating Emotional Regulation: The journey toward emotional mastery begins with the cultivation of emotional regulation.

Parents, by honing their ability to recognize and manage anger triggers, empower themselves to respond to challenging situations with equanimity. This, in turn, creates a ripple effect, fostering emotional regulation within the family unit.

2. Fostering Emotional Safety: A home characterized by effective anger management becomes a haven of emotional safety. Children, feeling secure in the predictability of emotional responses, develop a foundation for their own emotional well-being. The creation of this emotional safety net requires a commitment to ongoing self-reflection and growth.

3. Repairing and Strengthening Bonds: Acknowledging the emotional impact of explosive anger opens the door to repairing and strengthening parent-child bonds. Engaging in open and honest communication, parents can bridge the emotional gaps, fostering connections built on trust, understanding, and mutual respect.

The Journey to Mastery

Becoming the master of one's emotions is not an endpoint but a continuous journey of self-discovery and refinement. It involves a commitment to ongoing self-awareness, a willingness to seek support when needed, and a dedication to creating an emotionally nurturing environment for both oneself and one's children.

In subsequent chapters, we will delve deeper into practical strategies for recognizing and managing triggers, exploring the roots of explosive anger, and building a foundation for sustained emotional mastery. The journey toward becoming the master of your emotions is a courageous exploration that holds the promise of not only transforming your internal world but also shaping a future of emotional well-being for your entire family.

1.1.2 Behavioral Consequences

Understanding the intricacies of explosive anger goes beyond its emotional impact, extending into the realm of behavioral consequences. In the complex tapestry of parent-child relationships, the behavioral manifestations of parental anger are like threads that weave into the fabric of a child's development. This exploration seeks to illuminate the multifaceted dimensions of behavioral consequences, emphasizing the transformative potential of effective anger management. By mastering their emotions, parents embark on a journey to reshape not only their own behavior but also to foster an environment where positive behavioral patterns can flourish.

The Complex Weave of Behavioral Manifestations

Explosive anger in parents often leaves an imprint on the behavioral landscape within the family unit. These behavioral consequences, ranging from internalized struggles to outward expressions, have a profound impact on the child's development and the overall familial dynamic.

1. Internalized Effects: Children exposed to explosive anger may internalize the behavioral consequences, resulting in a myriad of challenges. Low self-esteem, feelings of inadequacy, and a distorted self-image can emerge as a direct result of the internalization of parental anger. This internal struggle may hinder the child's ability to navigate relationships and challenges in a healthy manner.

2. Externalized Behaviors: On the external front, behavioral consequences may manifest as defiant or aggressive actions. The child, lacking the emotional tools to process the intensity of parental anger, may externalize their distress through challenging behaviors. These outward expressions can create a cycle of frustration for both the child and the parent, further exacerbating the challenges within the family dynamic.

Academic and Cognitive Ramifications

The impact of explosive anger transcends the emotional and behavioral spheres, extending into the realm of academic performance and cognitive development. The child's ability to concentrate, learn, and engage in the learning process may be compromised due to the ongoing stress caused by the unpredictable nature of parental anger.

1. Academic Performance: The emotional turmoil resulting from parental anger can impede a child's focus and concentration. Academic performance may suffer, with grades reflecting the cognitive and emotional challenges faced by the child. The long-term consequences of academic struggles can affect the child's self-confidence and future educational pursuits.

2. Cognitive Development: A child's cognitive development is intricately linked

to their emotional well-being. Chronic exposure to explosive anger can hinder the development of cognitive skills such as problem-solving, decision-making, and critical thinking. The cognitive repercussions may echo into adulthood, influencing the child's ability to navigate the complexities of life.

The Role of Anger Management

Recognizing the behavioral consequences of explosive anger underscores the urgency of cultivating effective anger management strategies. By becoming the master of their emotions, parents not only break the cycle of negative behavioral patterns but also pave the way for positive, constructive interactions within the family.

1. Modeling Healthy Behavior: Parents serve as primary role models for their children. By mastering their own emotions and demonstrating healthy anger management, parents impart invaluable

lessons on constructive behavior. This modeling becomes the foundation upon which children build their own behavioral responses to stress and challenges.

2. Encouraging Emotional Expression: Effective anger management involves not only controlling the outward expression of anger but also encouraging healthy emotional expression. Creating an environment where emotions are acknowledged and expressed in a constructive manner fosters open communication and paves the way for a more positive behavioral atmosphere within the family.

3. Setting Boundaries with Consistency: Consistency in setting and enforcing boundaries is a fundamental aspect of effective anger management. Children thrive in environments where expectations are clear, and consequences are consistently applied. This approach provides a sense of security, reducing the likelihood of externalized behavioral challenges.

Cultivating Positive Behavioral Patterns

The journey toward mastering one's emotions and reshaping behavioral consequences is a nuanced process that requires commitment, self-reflection, and a willingness to embrace change. Parents, by undertaking this transformative journey, not only enhance their own well-being but also contribute to the creation of a home environment characterized by positive behavioral patterns.

In the forthcoming chapters, we will delve deeper into practical strategies for recognizing and managing triggers, understanding the roots of explosive anger, and building a foundation for sustained behavioral transformation. The mastery of emotions becomes not only a personal endeavor but a gift that reverberates through generations, shaping a legacy of resilience, understanding, and positive behavioral patterns within the family unit.

1.2 Impact on Family Dynamics

In the intricate tapestry of family life, the reverberations of explosive parental anger extend far beyond the individual, casting a profound shadow on the dynamics within the household. Family dynamics, shaped by the emotional climate set by parents, are crucial in determining the overall well-being of each family member. This exploration aims to unravel the intricate threads of how anger, when uncontrolled, can impact family dynamics and emphasizes the transformative potential of mastering one's emotions in fostering a harmonious familial environment.

The Ripple Effect on Family Relationships

Explosive anger disrupts the delicate balance within the family, creating a ripple effect that touches every member. The dynamics between parents, parent-child relationships, and sibling interactions are all influenced by the emotional turbulence stemming from unmanaged anger.

1. Parental Relationships: The relationship between parents is a cornerstone of family dynamics. Explosive anger can strain this vital connection, leading to communication breakdowns, emotional distance, and a general deterioration of spousal bonds. The spillover effect from one parent's anger onto the marital relationship can create a tense atmosphere that permeates the entire household.

2. Parent-Child Relationships: Parental anger casts a long shadow over parent-child relationships. The child, often caught in the crossfire, may experience confusion, fear, and a sense of instability. The establishment of a secure attachment, crucial for a child's emotional development, is hindered when explosive anger becomes a recurring theme within the family.

3. Sibling Interactions: Sibling relationships are not immune to the impact of explosive anger. The emotional climate within the family can affect how siblings relate to each other. Sibling conflicts may intensify as a result of the heightened stress and tension, further contributing to an emotionally charged family environment.

Shaping the Family Atmosphere

The emotional tone set by parents becomes the backdrop against which daily life unfolds for every family member. Unchecked anger can shape the family atmosphere in ways that hinder growth, communication, and the establishment of a nurturing home environment.

1. Communication Breakdown: Effective communication is the lifeblood of healthy family dynamics. Explosive anger disrupts this essential aspect, leading to communication breakdowns characterized by misunderstandings, emotional withdrawal, and a lack of open dialogue.

Rebuilding the bridges of communication requires a commitment to anger management and effective conflict resolution.

2. Emotional Instability: A family constantly navigating the storm of explosive anger becomes characterized by emotional instability. Children, in particular, may find it challenging to develop a sense of emotional security when the prevailing atmosphere is marked by unpredictability. Mastering emotions is thus not only a personal endeavor but a commitment to cultivating emotional stability within the family unit.

The Role of Anger Management in Family Harmony

Recognizing the impact of explosive anger on family dynamics underscores the urgency of effective anger management. By becoming the master of their emotions, parents take a significant step toward reshaping the family atmosphere and fostering harmony within the household.

1. Creating Emotional Safety: A home characterized by effective anger management becomes a sanctuary of emotional safety. Children, feeling secure in the predictability of emotional responses, can develop a sense of stability that contributes to their overall emotional well-being. Emotional safety is the bedrock upon which healthy family dynamics can be built.

2. Fostering Open Communication: Anger management is intricately linked to open communication. By mastering their emotions, parents create an environment where family members feel free to express themselves without fear of explosive reactions. This fosters a culture of open dialogue, enabling family members to navigate conflicts constructively.

3. Building Stronger Connections: The mastery of emotions paves the way for building stronger connections within the family. Parent-child relationships, sibling interactions, and spousal bonds can thrive in an environment characterized by understanding, empathy, and effective conflict resolution. This, in turn, shapes a family dynamic that nurtures the growth and well-being of each member.

The Journey to Family Well-being

The journey toward mastering one's emotions and reshaping family dynamics is a courageous undertaking that requires commitment, self-awareness, and a genuine desire for positive change. Parents, by undertaking this transformative journey, not only enhance their own well-being but contribute to the creation of a family environment characterized by love, understanding, and resilience.

In the forthcoming chapters, we will delve deeper into practical strategies for recognizing and managing triggers, understanding the roots of explosive anger, and building a foundation for sustained transformation within the family. The mastery of emotions becomes not only a personal endeavor but a legacy that shapes the dynamics of generations to come, fostering a home filled with harmony, understanding, and enduring familial connections.

1.3 Long-Term Consequences

In the intricate tapestry of family life, the repercussions of explosive parental anger are not confined to the immediate aftermath but reverberate through time, casting a shadow over the long-term well-being of both parents and children. This exploration delves into the nuanced dimensions of long-term consequences, emphasizing the transformative potential of mastering one's emotions in mitigating the enduring impact on familial relationships.

The Enduring Impact on Parent-Child Relationships

Parental anger, when left unmanaged, has the potential to shape the trajectory of parent-child relationships well into the future. The enduring consequences are multifaceted, influencing the emotional, psychological, and relational aspects of a child's development.

1. Interpersonal Relationships: Children raised in an environment marked by explosive anger may encounter challenges in forming and maintaining healthy interpersonal relationships. Trust issues, difficulty expressing emotions, and challenges in resolving conflicts amicably can persist into adulthood, impacting the quality of friendships, romantic relationships, and professional interactions.

2. Emotional Regulation: The ability to regulate emotions is a crucial life skill that influences various facets of adult life. Children exposed to unmanaged anger may face difficulties in developing effective emotional regulation strategies, leading to challenges in managing stress, navigating workplace dynamics, and fostering a sense of overall well-being.

The Impact on Academic and Professional Pursuits

The repercussions of explosive parental anger extend beyond the emotional and relational domains, influencing a child's academic and professional pursuits. The enduring consequences can manifest in various ways, hindering the individual's potential for success.

1. Academic Performance: The emotional distress caused by explosive anger can impede a child's ability to concentrate, learn, and perform academically. The enduring

impact may manifest in lower academic achievement, limited educational pursuits, and a potential reluctance to engage in lifelong learning.

2. Professional Relationships: The long-term consequences of unmanaged parental anger can extend into the professional realm. Difficulties in managing stress, conflicts, and emotions may impact the individual's ability to navigate workplace relationships, hindering career advancement and job satisfaction.

Shaping Patterns of Parenting

The enduring impact of parental anger is not isolated to the children alone but has a cyclical nature that can influence parenting styles in subsequent generations. Unresolved issues from childhood may resurface when individuals become parents themselves, perpetuating patterns of unmanaged anger.

1. Generational Patterns: The cycle of explosive anger may perpetuate through generations if not addressed. Adults who were exposed to unmanaged anger as children may inadvertently replicate similar patterns in their own parenting styles. Breaking free from generational patterns requires a commitment to self-awareness and intentional efforts toward emotional mastery.

2. Impact on Parental Well-being: The enduring consequences of unmanaged anger also affect the well-being of parents. Guilt, remorse, and unresolved emotional issues may linger, influencing mental health, self-esteem, and overall life satisfaction. The journey toward mastering emotions becomes not only a gift to the current generation but an investment in the well-being of future generations.

The Transformative Power of Anger Management

Recognizing the potential long-term consequences of explosive parental anger underscores the critical importance of effective anger management. By becoming the master of their emotions, parents embark on a transformative journey that not only mitigates the enduring impact on their children but also shapes a legacy of resilience, emotional intelligence, and familial well-being.

1. Breaking Generational Patterns: The mastery of emotions breaks the cycle of generational patterns, offering a new narrative for the family. Parents who engage in effective anger management become powerful agents of change, shaping a legacy characterized by healthier emotional dynamics and more constructive ways of relating to one another.

2. Cultivating Emotional Intelligence: Emotional intelligence, the ability to understand and manage one's own emotions and those of others, is a cornerstone of long-term well-being. Parents who master

their emotions model and cultivate emotional intelligence within the family, providing children with essential tools for navigating the complexities of life.

The Lifelong Journey of Emotional Mastery

The journey toward mastering one's emotions and mitigating the long-term consequences of parental anger is a lifelong endeavor. It involves a commitment to ongoing self-awareness, a willingness to seek support when needed, and a dedication to creating a familial environment characterized by understanding, love, and enduring emotional well-being.

In subsequent chapters, we will delve deeper into practical strategies for recognizing and managing triggers, understanding the roots of explosive anger, and building a foundation for sustained emotional transformation. The mastery of emotions becomes not only a personal endeavor but a legacy that shapes the dynamics of generations to come, fostering a home filled with resilience, understanding, and enduring familial connections.

Chapter 2: Recognizing Your Triggers

2.1 Identifying Personal Triggers

In the intricate landscape of mastering one's emotions, a crucial and transformative step is the identification of personal triggers. Triggers are the catalysts that ignite the flames of anger, and understanding them is paramount for effective anger management, especially for parents striving to be the masters of their emotions. This chapter delves into the nuanced process of identifying personal triggers, recognizing their origins, and laying the foundation for constructive and intentional responses.

The Nature of Personal Triggers

Personal triggers are unique emotional landmines that, when activated, lead to heightened emotional responses, particularly anger. Identifying these triggers requires a deep dive into one's emotional landscape and an honest exploration of past experiences and present stressors.

1. Past Experiences: Triggers often find their roots in past experiences, especially those that were emotionally charged or traumatic. Unresolved issues from childhood, relationship dynamics, or personal traumas can become triggers when similar situations arise, leading to an outpouring of anger as a defense mechanism.

2. Present Stressors: Current stressors, whether related to work, finances, or interpersonal relationships, can serve as triggers. The cumulative effect of daily stressors can lower the threshold for emotional reactions, making it easier for minor incidents to elicit an outsized anger response.

The Importance of Self-Reflection

Identifying personal triggers is an introspective process that demands self-reflection and a willingness to confront uncomfortable aspects of one's emotional landscape. This self-awareness lays the groundwork for proactive and intentional anger management.

1. Journaling and Reflection: Maintaining a journal to record instances of anger, the associated emotions, and the circumstances leading to the emotional response can be a powerful tool. Regular reflection on these entries helps uncover patterns and identify recurring triggers.

2. Therapeutic Support: Seeking the guidance of a mental health professional can provide invaluable insights. Therapists can assist in navigating the complexities of one's emotional triggers, offering a safe space for exploration and equipping individuals with coping mechanisms.

Uncovering Patterns and Themes

Identifying personal triggers involves recognizing patterns and themes that emerge across various situations. These patterns can reveal deeper emotional wounds or unresolved issues that contribute to the intensity of anger responses.

1. Common Situational Factors: Observing commonalities in triggering situations is key. Are certain themes, environments, or types of interactions consistently leading to anger? Identifying these common factors sheds light on specific triggers that require attention.

2. Emotional Themes: Beyond external circumstances, emotional themes play a significant role. Are feelings of inadequacy, fear, or frustration consistently associated with anger episodes? Understanding the emotional undercurrents provides insight into the root causes of triggered responses.

Transformative Strategies for Trigger Management

Once personal triggers are identified, the journey toward mastery involves developing strategies for trigger management. These strategies empower parents to respond consciously rather than reactively, fostering a more harmonious emotional environment within the family.

1. Mindfulness Practices: Cultivating mindfulness through practices such as meditation, deep breathing, or yoga enhances emotional awareness. Mindfulness allows individuals to observe their thoughts and emotions without immediate reaction, providing a buffer against impulsive anger responses.

2. Cognitive Restructuring: Cognitive restructuring involves challenging and reframing negative thought patterns associated with triggers. By consciously changing the narrative and adopting a more balanced perspective, parents can alter their emotional responses to triggering situations.

3. Communication Skills: Developing effective communication skills is pivotal in trigger management. Expressing feelings assertively, actively listening to others, and choosing words carefully contribute to creating an open and constructive dialogue, minimizing the potential for triggered anger.

The Ongoing Journey of Emotional Mastery

Identifying personal triggers marks a significant milestone on the path to emotional mastery, but the journey is ongoing. It involves a commitment to continuous self-reflection, the implementation of learned strategies, and an openness to adapting and refining approaches as needed.

1. Embracing Growth and Adaptation: The ability to adapt and grow in response to

identified triggers is essential. Life circumstances change, and so do personal dynamics. Being open to evolving strategies and embracing personal growth contributes to sustained emotional mastery.

2. Modeling Emotional Intelligence: Parents who actively engage in the process of identifying and managing triggers become powerful role models for their children. Modeling emotional intelligence and proactive anger management sets the stage for healthier emotional responses within the family.

In the realm of parental anger management, identifying personal triggers lays a foundational cornerstone for lasting emotional well-being. It empowers parents to navigate the complexities of family life with intentionality, fostering an environment characterized by understanding, patience, and resilience. The ongoing commitment to self-reflection and trigger management becomes not only a personal journey but a transformative gift to the entire family.

2.1.1 Reflecting on Past Incidents

The journey towards mastering one's emotions, especially in the context of parental anger management, involves a significant aspect of reflecting on past incidents. This reflective process serves as a catalyst for personal growth, offering valuable insights into patterns, triggers, and the emotional landscape. In this chapter, we explore the importance of reflecting on past incidents, the transformative power it holds, and how it contributes to building a foundation for healthier emotional responses.

Unveiling Patterns through Reflection

Reflecting on past incidents provides a lens through which individuals can examine recurring patterns in their emotional responses. It is an opportunity to dissect the dynamics of anger, understand the factors that contribute to its escalation, and recognize the patterns that may be hindering emotional well-being.

1. Identifying Triggers: Past incidents often serve as clues to underlying triggers. By revisiting moments of heightened anger, individuals can identify the specific circumstances, words, or actions that acted as catalysts. This awareness is fundamental to effective trigger management.

2. Examining Emotional Responses: Reflecting on past incidents allows for an examination of the emotional responses associated with anger. Were there consistent themes of frustration, disappointment, or fear? Understanding the underlying emotions provides a roadmap for addressing core issues.

The Role of Self-Compassion

Reflection on past incidents should be approached with self-compassion. It's an acknowledgment that everyone is a work in progress, and growth often emerges from moments of vulnerability. Self-compassion during reflection allows individuals to learn from their experiences without succumbing to guilt or self-blame.

1. Learning from Mistakes: Mistakes are inherent to the human experience. Reflecting on past incidents is an opportunity to learn from these mistakes, gaining wisdom that contributes to personal and emotional growth. It's not about dwelling on faults but leveraging them for positive change.

2. Cultivating Forgiveness: Reflective practices should include an element of self-forgiveness. Holding onto guilt or resentment towards oneself can impede growth. Cultivating forgiveness creates space for healing and encourages a forward-looking perspective.

Gaining Emotional Intelligence

Reflection on past incidents is a gateway to developing emotional intelligence. Emotional intelligence involves recognizing, understanding, and managing one's own emotions, and it forms the cornerstone of effective anger management.

1. Recognizing Emotional Triggers: Through reflection, individuals can refine their ability to recognize emotional triggers in real-time. This heightened awareness empowers them to implement coping strategies and respond more skillfully to challenging situations.

2. Understanding Emotional Impact: Examining the aftermath of past incidents allows for an understanding of the emotional impact on oneself and others. This understanding fosters empathy, a crucial

component of emotional intelligence, and encourages the cultivation of healthier emotional dynamics.

Strategies for Reflective Practice

Incorporating reflective practices into daily life is essential for ongoing personal growth in anger management. These strategies are adaptable and can be tailored to individual preferences and lifestyles.

1. Journaling: Keeping a reflective journal provides a structured space to document emotions, triggers, and insights from past incidents. Regular journaling creates a tangible record of progress and facilitates the identification of patterns.

2. Mindfulness Meditation: Mindfulness meditation encourages staying present in the moment without judgment. Incorporating mindfulness into daily routines enhances the ability to reflect on past incidents with

clarity and without being overwhelmed by emotions.

3. Seeking Feedback: Engaging in open and honest conversations with trusted friends, family members, or a mental health professional can provide valuable external perspectives. Others may offer insights that individuals might overlook in self-reflection.

The Transformative Power of Reflection

Reflecting on past incidents is not merely a retrospective exercise; it is a transformative journey that shapes the present and future. It allows individuals to consciously choose how they respond to similar situations, fostering a proactive and intentional approach to anger management.

1. Empowering Proactive Responses: Armed with insights from reflective practices, individuals gain the power to respond proactively to triggers. The ability to pause, assess, and choose a measured response is a

testament to the transformative impact of reflection.

2. Building Resilience: Reflection contributes to the development of emotional resilience. Learning from past incidents, understanding personal triggers, and implementing effective coping strategies create a foundation for navigating future challenges with greater ease and resilience.

In the tapestry of mastering one's emotions and managing anger, reflecting on past incidents is not a one-time endeavor but a continuous journey of growth. It is a commitment to self-awareness, a testament to resilience, and a pathway to building emotional intelligence. By embracing the transformative power of reflection, individuals embark on a journey that transcends the limitations of past incidents, creating a future characterized by emotional mastery and well-being.

2.1.2 Common Triggers for Parents

In the intricate dance of parenting, understanding and managing triggers is a cornerstone of effective anger management. Triggers are the subtle or overt stimuli that can evoke intense emotional responses, often leading to anger. This chapter explores common triggers for parents, unraveling the complexities that lie beneath the surface. By identifying and addressing these triggers, parents can navigate the path to emotional mastery and foster a more harmonious family environment.

The Juggling Act of Parenting

Parenting is a multifaceted role that requires constant adaptation and resilience. The demands of balancing work, household responsibilities, and the intricate dynamics of family life can create a pressure cooker of stress, making parents susceptible to specific triggers.

1. Work-Life Balance: The delicate equilibrium between professional responsibilities and family life is a common trigger. The stressors of work, coupled with the desire to be present for one's children, can create a volatile emotional landscape. Striking a harmonious work-life balance is crucial for mitigating this trigger.

2. Fatigue and Sleep Deprivation: Parenting often entails interrupted sleep patterns, especially in the early years. The cumulative effects of fatigue and sleep deprivation can lower the threshold for emotional resilience, making parents more susceptible to irritability and frustration.

Emotional Dynamics within the Family

The intricate dance of family dynamics introduces a myriad of triggers, emanating from the relationships between parents and their children or among siblings.

1. Sibling Conflicts: The inevitable conflicts between siblings can act as potent triggers for parents. Constant bickering, disagreements, or the need to mediate disputes can contribute to elevated stress levels, testing the emotional resilience of parents.

2. Challenges in Parent-Child Communication: Miscommunication or a lack of understanding between parents and their children can be a significant trigger. The frustration of not being able to convey expectations or comprehend the needs of a child can lead to heightened emotional responses.

Personal Stressors and Triggers

Beyond the realm of parenting, personal stressors and unresolved issues from the past can serve as powerful triggers, influencing emotional responses within the family dynamic.

1. Financial Strain: Economic challenges or financial strain can amplify stress levels for parents. The pressure to provide for the family's needs and aspirations can contribute to feelings of inadequacy and frustration.

2. Unresolved Personal Issues: Parents bring their own histories and experiences into the realm of parenting. Unresolved personal issues, whether related to relationships, past traumas, or unfulfilled aspirations, can become triggers when intersecting with the challenges of parenting.

Unrealistic Expectations and Societal Pressures

Societal expectations and the pressure to conform to idealized standards of parenting can create an additional layer of triggers for parents.

1. Comparisons and Judgment: The pervasive culture of comparing one's parenting style or children's achievements to

others can breed insecurity and trigger feelings of inadequacy. The fear of judgment from peers or societal standards can add an extra layer of stress.

2. Cultural or Gender Expectations: Cultural or gender-based expectations can also act as triggers. Striving to fulfill prescribed roles or expectations may lead to internal conflicts, especially if they clash with an individual's values or desires.

Strategies for Trigger Management

Identifying common triggers is a crucial step, but effective anger management requires strategies for navigating these triggers proactively.

1. Self-Care Practices: Prioritizing self-care is fundamental. Adequate sleep, regular exercise, and moments of personal rejuvenation contribute to emotional resilience, reducing the impact of triggers.

2. Effective Communication: Improving communication within the family is a powerful strategy. Creating an open space for dialogue, active listening, and expressing emotions constructively fosters understanding and mitigates the potential for triggers.

3. Setting Realistic Expectations: Establishing realistic expectations for oneself as a parent and for the family as a whole is crucial. Embracing the imperfections of parenting and acknowledging that challenges are a natural part of the journey can alleviate the pressure that triggers may induce.

The Journey to Emotional Mastery

Navigating the common triggers for parents is an integral part of the journey towards emotional mastery. It involves a commitment to self-awareness, proactive strategies, and a willingness to adapt. By understanding the intricacies of these triggers, parents can transform challenges into opportunities for growth, ultimately fostering a home environment characterized by emotional intelligence, resilience, and genuine connection. The journey to emotional mastery is not without its twists and turns, but with dedication and a compassionate approach, parents can become true masters of their emotions, enriching both their lives and the lives of their children.

2.2 Recognizing Early Warning Signs

In the intricate tapestry of parenting, recognizing the early warning signs of escalating anger is akin to having a beacon that guides parents toward emotional mastery. This chapter explores the subtle cues and signals that precede heightened anger, providing insights into the importance of early recognition. By understanding these early warning signs, parents can proactively navigate the tumultuous seas of emotions, ultimately becoming the masters of their own reactions and fostering a more nurturing family environment.

The Unspoken Language of Emotions

Emotions often communicate through a language of their own, with early warning signs acting as silent messengers. Recognizing these signs requires a heightened level of self-awareness and attunement to one's emotional landscape.

1. Physical Cues: Physical manifestations often precede the eruption of anger. Tension in the shoulders, clenching fists, increased heart rate, or a feeling of heat rising are common physical cues. These subtle changes in the body serve as early indicators of heightened emotional arousal.

2. Changes in Breathing Patterns: The breath is intimately connected to emotional states. Shallow or rapid breathing can signal increasing stress levels. Recognizing changes in breathing patterns offers an

opportunity for intervention before emotions escalate further.

Emotional Precursors to Anger

Emotions are multi-faceted, and specific emotional states can act as precursors to anger. Understanding these emotional precursors allows parents to address underlying issues before anger takes center stage.

1. Frustration: Frustration often precedes anger. It is a signal that expectations or desires are not being met. Identifying moments of frustration enables parents to explore the root causes and address them proactively.

2. Feeling Overwhelmed: The demands of parenting can sometimes become overwhelming. When parents feel a sense of being inundated or stretched beyond capacity, it can set the stage for heightened emotional responses. Recognizing this

feeling of overwhelm is crucial for preventive measures.

Cognitive Warning Signs

The way we think about a situation can significantly impact our emotional responses. Cognitive warning signs involve patterns of thought that may indicate an impending escalation of anger.

1. Negative Thought Patterns:
Negative self-talk or thoughts about the situation can contribute to escalating anger. Recognizing the emergence of negative thought patterns provides an opportunity for cognitive restructuring before emotions intensify.

2. Rigid Thinking: A tendency towards rigid thinking or a refusal to consider alternative perspectives can fuel anger. Acknowledging when thoughts become inflexible allows parents to introduce adaptability and openness into their mindset.

Environmental Triggers

The context in which parenting unfolds can also serve as a trigger. Recognizing environmental factors that contribute to escalating emotions is pivotal for preemptive action.

1. Lack of Time or Privacy: A shortage of time or the absence of personal space can heighten stress levels. Acknowledging these environmental stressors allows parents to implement strategies such as time management or boundary-setting.

2. Unresolved Issues: Lingering unresolved issues, whether within the family or from external sources, can act as persistent triggers. Identifying these unresolved matters enables parents to address them in a timely and constructive manner.

The Power of Mindful Observation

Mindful observation involves cultivating a non-judgmental awareness of one's thoughts, feelings, and bodily sensations. This practice is a powerful tool for recognizing early warning signs, as it allows parents to observe their internal landscape without immediate reactivity.

1. Mindful Breathing: Incorporating mindful breathing exercises into daily routines enhances the ability to observe changes in breath patterns. Mindful breathing serves as an anchor, grounding parents in the present moment and fostering awareness of their emotional state.

2. Regular Self-Check-Ins: Implementing regular self-check-ins throughout the day encourages a conscious observation of emotional states. These brief moments of reflection empower parents to identify early warning signs and take preventive measures.

Strategies for Early Intervention

Recognizing early warning signs is the first step; the next involves implementing strategies for early intervention. Parents can develop a personalized toolkit of techniques to navigate emotional escalation effectively.

1. Pause and Reflect: Creating a habit of pausing and reflecting when early warning signs emerge provides a buffer before emotional escalation. This momentary pause allows parents to assess the situation and choose a measured response.

2. Implement Stress-Reduction Techniques: Integrating stress-reduction techniques, such as deep breathing, meditation, or physical activity, into daily life can mitigate the impact of early warning signs. These techniques serve as proactive measures to maintain emotional balance.

3. Communication Strategies: Establishing clear communication channels within the family is essential. When early warning signs arise, effective communication,

including expressing feelings assertively and actively listening, becomes a valuable tool for resolution.

The Journey to Emotional Mastery

Recognizing early warning signs is a pivotal component of the journey to emotional mastery in parenting. It involves a commitment to self-awareness, mindful observation, and the implementation of proactive strategies for intervention. By understanding the unspoken language of emotions, parents become adept at navigating the nuanced landscape of parenting, fostering a home environment characterized by emotional intelligence, resilience, and genuine connection. The journey to emotional mastery is a continuous process, and with each recognition of early warning signs, parents take another step toward creating a nurturing and harmonious family dynamic.

2.2.1 Physical Signals

In the intricate dance of parental anger management, the body often becomes a silent narrator, conveying the unspoken language of emotions through physical signals. Recognizing these cues is akin to deciphering a crucial code on the path to emotional mastery. This chapter delves into the nuanced realm of physical signals, exploring the intricate ways in which the body communicates impending anger. By understanding and addressing these physical signals, parents can navigate the complex seas of emotions with greater awareness, ultimately becoming the masters of their own emotional responses and fostering a more harmonious family environment.

The Body's Silent Symphony

The body's response to emotions is orchestrated by a symphony of physiological changes. Recognizing the subtle notes of this silent symphony allows parents to intervene before anger crescendos into uncontrolled emotional outbursts.

1. Muscle Tension: One of the earliest physical signals is muscle tension. A tightening in the shoulders, neck, or jaw can signify mounting stress. Parents attuned to these physical cues can employ relaxation techniques to alleviate tension before it transforms into anger.

2. Clenched Fists: The simple act of clenching fists can be an unconscious response to building anger. This physical manifestation is a precursor to heightened emotional arousal and serves as a clear indicator for parents to pause, reflect, and intervene.

The Breath as a Barometer

The breath, intricately connected to emotional states, serves as a barometer for the body's response to stress and anger. Understanding changes in breathing patterns is pivotal in early intervention.

1. Shallow Breathing: As stress levels rise, breathing may become shallower. This physiological response limits the flow of oxygen, contributing to heightened emotional arousal. Parents who recognize shallow breathing can employ deep-breathing exercises to restore calm.

2. Rapid Breathing: An acceleration in breathing rate is a common sign of escalating emotions. Rapid breathing contributes to a heightened state of physiological arousal, making it essential for parents to identify and regulate their breath to prevent emotional escalation.

Temperature Changes

The body's temperature can undergo subtle shifts in response to emotional arousal. Recognizing these changes provides valuable insights into the body's physical response to stress and anger.

1. Feeling Warm or Flushed: An increase in body temperature, leading to a warm or flushed sensation, is a common physical signal. This can be an early indicator of heightened stress levels. Parents attuned to this change can take proactive measures to cool down both physically and emotionally.

2. Cold Sensations: Conversely, some individuals may experience a sensation of coldness or chills as a response to stress. Recognizing these temperature shifts allows parents to address the physiological aspects of anger before it intensifies.

Gastrointestinal Distress

The gut-brain connection is a well-established aspect of emotional physiology. Gastrointestinal distress can manifest as a physical signal of mounting stress and anger.

1. Butterflies or Nausea: The sensation of butterflies in the stomach or nausea can

accompany emotional turmoil. Parents who notice these gastrointestinal signals can take steps to address the root causes of stress, preventing the escalation of negative emotions.

2. Digestive Discomfort: Stress and anger can contribute to digestive discomfort, such as stomach cramps or indigestion. Recognizing these physical manifestations prompts parents to engage in self-care practices that promote both emotional and digestive well-being.

Strategies for Physical Signal Management

Understanding physical signals is the first step; the next involves implementing strategies for effective management. Parents can develop a toolkit of techniques to address physical signals and prevent the escalation of anger.

1. Body Scan Meditation: Incorporating body scan meditation into daily routines fosters awareness of physical sensations. This mindfulness practice enables parents to detect subtle changes and intervene before physical signals intensify.

2. Progressive Muscle Relaxation: Progressive muscle relaxation is a technique that involves systematically tensing and then releasing muscle groups. This practice promotes overall relaxation and helps alleviate tension, addressing one of the earliest physical signals of anger.

3. Breathing Exercises: Implementing breathing exercises, such as diaphragmatic breathing or box breathing, allows parents to regulate their breath and counteract changes in breathing patterns. These exercises serve as powerful tools for emotional regulation.

Navigating the intricate landscape of parental anger management involves recognizing and interpreting the body's silent symphony of physical signals. By understanding the language of muscle tension, breath patterns, temperature changes, and gastrointestinal distress, parents gain valuable insights into the early warning signs of anger. The journey toward emotional mastery becomes a symphony of self-regulation, where parents harmonize with the body's cues to intervene proactively. In doing so, they cultivate an environment characterized by emotional intelligence, resilience, and authentic connections within the family. The mastery of physical signals becomes not only a personal endeavor but a transformative gift that enriches the entire family dynamic.

2.2.2 Emotional Cues

In the intricate realm of parental anger management, emotions play a symphony of cues, revealing the subtle nuances of internal states. Decoding emotional cues is akin to wielding a compass that guides parents through the labyrinth of their feelings, offering an opportunity for self-awareness and proactive intervention. This chapter delves into the intricacies of emotional cues, exploring the varied signals that precede heightened anger. By understanding and navigating these emotional cues, parents can become the masters of their emotional responses, fostering a more serene and connected family environment.

The Language of Emotions

Emotions serve as messengers, conveying valuable information about one's internal state. Recognizing and interpreting this emotional language is fundamental in the journey toward parental anger management.

1. Irritability and Frustration: Irritability and frustration are early emotional cues that often precede anger. These emotions signal a perceived obstacle or challenge, serving as a call to attention. Parents who acknowledge these cues can intervene before frustration transforms into uncontrolled anger.

2.   Increased   Sensitivity: Heightened sensitivity to stimuli, whether noise, comments, or actions, is a notable emotional cue. This increased sensitivity can indicate emotional vulnerability, prompting parents to engage in self-care or seek support before heightened anger ensues.

Patterns of Thought and Interpretation

The way parents interpret situations and their thought patterns contribute significantly to emotional cues. Understanding these cognitive aspects allows for targeted intervention.

1. Negative Self-Talk: Negative self-talk or internal dialogue that magnifies stressors can act as a precursor to anger. Recognizing and challenging negative thoughts enables parents to alter their mental landscape, preventing the escalation of anger.

2. Catastrophizing: Catastrophizing involves anticipating the worst possible outcome in a given situation. This cognitive pattern heightens stress levels and can contribute to anger. Parents who identify this tendency can adopt a more balanced perspective, mitigating the emotional impact.

Changes in Mood and Energy

Shifts in mood and energy levels are tangible indicators of emotional cues. Recognizing these shifts allows parents to address underlying emotions before they intensify.

1. Sudden Changes in Mood: Abrupt shifts from a positive to a negative mood may signify underlying emotional turbulence. Identifying these changes prompts parents to explore the root causes and implement strategies for emotional regulation.

2. Low Energy and Motivation: A decline in energy and motivation can be a sign of

emotional fatigue. When parents recognize these cues, they can prioritize self-care to replenish emotional reserves and prevent the onset of anger.

Emotional Resonance with Past Experiences

Emotional cues often resonate with past experiences, serving as echoes of unresolved emotions. Understanding this resonance provides insight into deeper emotional currents.

1. Flashbacks or Intrusive Memories: Flashbacks or intrusive memories related to past experiences can evoke intense emotions. Parents who recognize these emotional cues can engage in self-compassion and seek therapeutic support to address underlying issues.

2. Triggers from Childhood: Certain situations may act as triggers, resonating with unresolved emotions from childhood.

Identifying these triggers allows parents to separate past experiences from present circumstances and respond with greater emotional intelligence.

Strategies for Emotional Cue Navigation

Decoding emotional cues is a valuable skill, and parents can employ various strategies for effective navigation and intervention.

1. Mindfulness Practices: Mindfulness involves being fully present in the current moment. Practices such as mindfulness meditation or mindful breathing enhance awareness of emotional cues, enabling parents to respond consciously rather than reactively.

2. Emotional Journaling: Maintaining an emotional journal provides a structured outlet for expressing and reflecting on emotions. Regular journaling enhances self-awareness and allows parents to track patterns of emotional cues over time.

3. Therapeutic Support: Seeking the guidance of a mental health professional offers a supportive space for exploring emotional cues and developing coping strategies. Therapy can be instrumental in addressing deeper emotional currents and fostering resilience.

The Transformative Power of Emotional Mastery

In the intricate dance of decoding emotional cues, parents embark on a transformative journey toward emotional mastery. By understanding the language of irritability, shifts in mood, cognitive patterns, and emotional resonance, parents gain insight into the subtleties of their internal landscape. The mastery of emotional cues becomes a compass, guiding parents toward self-awareness, resilience, and the capacity to respond to challenging situations with emotional intelligence.

Decoding emotional cues is a symphony of self-understanding, where each note represents an opportunity for growth and intervention. In the realm of parental anger management, this skill becomes not only a personal endeavor but a gift to the entire family. By navigating the intricate nuances of emotional cues, parents lay the foundation for a home environment characterized by connection, empathy, and a profound mastery of emotions. The journey is ongoing, and with each decoded cue, parents inch closer to creating a harmonious family dynamic that reflects the transformative power of emotional mastery.

Chapter 3: Understanding the Roots of Anger

3.1 Exploring Childhood Influences

In the intricate tapestry of parental anger management, the exploration of childhood influences serves as a compass, guiding parents to the roots of their emotional responses. This chapter delves into the profound impact of early experiences on the development of anger management skills. By unraveling the threads of childhood influences, parents can gain a deeper understanding of their emotional landscape, ultimately empowering themselves to be the masters of their emotions and create a more harmonious family environment.

The Echoes of Early Experiences

Childhood experiences form the foundation of emotional responses in adulthood. Exploring these influences unveils the echoes of past interactions, shaping the lens through which parents perceive and manage anger.

1. Modeling Behavior: Children absorb behavior by observing their caregivers. If parents witnessed uncontrolled anger during their upbringing, they may unconsciously replicate these patterns. Recognizing and addressing these learned behaviors is pivotal in breaking the cycle.

2. Communication Styles: The way emotions, particularly anger, were communicated in the family of origin influences a parent's communication style. An environment where anger was expressed explosively or repressed can impact how parents navigate and express their emotions.

Unresolved Childhood Trauma

Childhood trauma, whether overt or subtle, can cast a long shadow on emotional well-being. Exploring these unresolved traumas is a courageous step in the journey toward parental anger management.

1. Impact of Abuse or Neglect: Experiences of abuse or neglect during childhood can leave enduring emotional imprints. Unresolved trauma may manifest as anger, and parents who recognize these echoes can seek therapeutic support to heal and break the cycle.

2. Attachment Patterns: Attachment patterns established in early relationships significantly influence how individuals regulate emotions. Insecure attachments may contribute to heightened emotional responses, emphasizing the importance of understanding and addressing these patterns.

Parenting Styles and Beliefs

The parenting styles experienced during childhood contribute to the formation of beliefs about emotions and their expression. Exploring these influences provides insight into one's approach to parenting and anger management.

1. Authoritarian vs. Permissive Styles: Individuals raised in authoritarian environments may internalize a sense of powerlessness, leading to frustration and explosive anger. Conversely, permissive parenting may result in difficulties establishing boundaries, contributing to anger arising from perceived chaos.

2. Cultural and Societal Beliefs: Cultural and societal beliefs surrounding anger and its expression shape parental attitudes. Understanding the cultural context in which anger was addressed during childhood aids in dismantling potentially limiting beliefs and adopting healthier approaches.

Self-Reflection and Personal Growth

Exploring childhood influences is a journey of self-reflection and personal growth. It involves a willingness to confront and understand the impact of early experiences on emotional responses.

1.   Journaling   and   Self-Reflection: Maintaining a journal allows parents to explore memories, emotions, and patterns from their childhood. Self-reflection enables individuals to identify connections between past experiences and present emotional responses.

2.   Therapeutic Support: Seeking the guidance of a mental health professional provides a safe space to explore childhood influences. Therapy allows individuals to process and make sense of their experiences, fostering emotional healing and growth.

Breaking Generational Patterns

For many parents, the exploration of childhood influences is not only a personal endeavor but a commitment to breaking generational patterns. It involves the conscious decision to cultivate a different emotional landscape for the next generation.

1. Intentional Parenting: Recognizing the impact of childhood influences empowers parents to be intentional in their approach to parenting. It involves making conscious choices to create an environment that fosters emotional intelligence, open communication, and healthy anger management.

2. Communication Skills: Developing effective communication skills is crucial in breaking generational patterns. By cultivating a family environment where emotions are openly discussed and understood, parents contribute to the dismantling of old paradigms.

Exploring childhood influences in the context of parental anger management is a journey of emotional liberation. It is a voyage that requires courage, self-reflection, and a commitment to personal growth. By unraveling the threads of early experiences, parents gain insights into the roots of their emotional responses and, in doing so, free themselves from the limitations of generational patterns. The journey is transformative, leading to emotional mastery and the creation of a family environment characterized by understanding, resilience, and the breaking of old chains. As parents navigate this intricate exploration, they not only liberate themselves but also pave the way for a legacy of emotional well-being for generations to come.

3.1.1 Examining Your Own Upbringing

In the intricate tapestry of parental anger management, examining one's own upbringing acts as a reflective mirror, revealing patterns, influences, and emotional imprints. This chapter delves into the profound impact of personal upbringing on the development of anger management skills. By scrutinizing the experiences, lessons, and dynamics of one's own upbringing, parents can embark on a transformative journey toward mastering their emotions and cultivating a more harmonious family environment.

Unraveling the Threads of Childhood Lessons

The lessons learned during childhood serve as a blueprint for emotional responses in adulthood. Examining one's upbringing involves unraveling the threads of these early lessons, shedding light on the origins of patterns and behaviors.

1. Observing Parental Models: Children often mirror the behaviors modeled by their parents. Examining the ways in which anger was expressed or managed in the parental home provides insight into learned patterns that may influence current parenting practices.

2. Impact of Discipline Strategies: Discipline strategies employed during

childhood contribute to the formation of beliefs about authority and consequences. Understanding the impact of disciplinary measures on one's emotional landscape informs the development of effective and mindful approaches to discipline as a parent.

Communication Styles and Expression of Emotions

The communication styles witnessed and experienced during upbringing significantly influence how individuals express and manage their emotions. Examining these styles provides a foundation for enhancing communication within the family.

1. Openness vs. Repression: Families vary in their approach to expressing emotions. Some cultivate an environment of openness, encouraging the free expression of feelings, while others may lean towards emotional repression. Understanding these dynamics shapes how parents navigate emotional conversations with their own children.

2. Conflict Resolution Models: The methods used to resolve conflicts within the family of origin impact how individuals approach conflict as parents. Examining these models allows for the identification of effective conflict resolution strategies and the abandonment of counterproductive patterns.

Emotional Impact of Upbringing on Beliefs and Values

The emotional impact of one's upbringing extends beyond behaviors and communication styles, influencing deeply held beliefs and values related to anger management.

1. Beliefs About Anger: The beliefs formed during childhood about the acceptability and expression of anger contribute to a parent's internal dialogue. Examining these beliefs allows for the identification of potentially limiting perspectives and the adoption of healthier attitudes toward anger.

2. Cultural and Familial Values: Cultural and familial values surrounding emotional expression shape the lens through which parents view anger. Understanding these values provides a nuanced perspective and the opportunity to navigate between cultural influences and personal beliefs.

Patterns to Retain and Those to Transform

The examination of one's upbringing involves a discerning look at patterns and practices that may be worth retaining and those that require transformation for effective anger management.

1. Positive Parenting Practices: Identifying positive parenting practices observed during upbringing offers a template for nurturing a supportive and loving family environment. Recognizing and retaining these practices contributes to a healthy emotional landscape.

2. Breaking Negative Patterns: Concurrently, recognizing negative patterns witnessed during childhood allows for intentional efforts to break these cycles. Examining and transforming counterproductive patterns ensure that parents do not inadvertently pass on harmful behaviors to the next generation.

Self-Compassion in the Process

The examination of one's upbringing requires a stance of self-compassion. It involves acknowledging that everyone is shaped by a combination of positive and challenging experiences, and growth is a continuous process.

1. Learning from Mistakes: Mistakes made by parents or caregivers during upbringing are part of the human experience. Examining these mistakes provides an opportunity to learn and grow, fostering resilience and an openness to self-improvement.

2. Cultivating Forgiveness: Examining one's upbringing also entails cultivating forgiveness, both for oneself and for those who played a role in shaping that experience. Letting go of resentment and blame creates space for emotional healing and personal growth.

Integrating Insights into Parental Practices

The examination of one's upbringing is not an end in itself but a means to integrate valuable insights into current parental practices. It involves a commitment to mindfulness, self-awareness, and the intentional shaping of a nurturing family environment.

1. Mindful Parenting: Mindful parenting is rooted in the awareness of the present moment and a non-judgmental acceptance of oneself and one's children. Examining one's upbringing contributes to the development of mindful parenting practices that prioritize

emotional intelligence and effective anger management.

2. Effective Communication Strategies: Integrating insights from the examination of one's upbringing into communication strategies ensures that parents create an environment where emotions are expressed openly, and conflicts are resolved constructively.

Examining one's own upbringing is a transformative journey that unfolds through self-reflection, self-compassion, and a commitment to personal growth. It is a pivotal step toward mastering one's emotions and creating a family environment characterized by understanding, resilience, and emotional intelligence. By holding the mirror to the past, parents not only gain insights into their own emotional landscape but also pave the way for a future where the echoes of positive influences surpass the limitations of the past, fostering a legacy of emotional well-being for generations to come.

3.1.2 Breaking Generational Patterns

In the intricate tapestry of parental anger management, breaking generational patterns is a courageous and transformative endeavor. This chapter delves into the profound significance of disrupting inherited cycles of anger expression, guiding parents on a liberating journey toward becoming the masters of their emotions. By consciously challenging and reshaping generational patterns, parents pave the way for a family dynamic characterized by understanding, resilience, and emotional intelligence.

The Inheritance of Emotional Legacies

Generational patterns of anger management are often inherited, passed down from one generation to the next. Understanding the roots of these patterns involves recognizing the emotional legacies that shape family dynamics.

1. Learned Behaviors: Behaviors related to anger are learned through observation and mimicry within the family. Parents may unintentionally pass down reactive patterns of anger expression, perpetuating a cycle that requires conscious intervention to break. 2. Cultural and Familial Norms: Cultural and familial norms around anger play a significant role. Whether expressing anger is deemed acceptable or repressed varies across cultures and families, influencing how parents navigate and model anger management.

The Decision to Break Free

Breaking generational patterns begins with a conscious decision to break free from ingrained habits and responses. It involves a commitment to chart a new course that prioritizes emotional well-being and healthy anger management.

1. Conscious Awareness: The first step is cultivating conscious awareness of the patterns inherited from past generations. This involves reflecting on one's own responses to anger and recognizing when reactions align with, or deviate from, the patterns observed in the family of origin.

2. Intentional Self-Reflection: Intentional self-reflection allows parents to delve into the deeper layers of their emotional responses. Exploring the reasons behind certain reactions provides insight into the generational influences shaping anger management styles.

Identifying Counterproductive Patterns

To break free from generational patterns, it is crucial to identify counterproductive patterns that hinder effective anger management. This involves acknowledging harmful behaviors and making a commitment to transformative change.

1. Explosive Outbursts: If explosive anger outbursts were commonplace in the family of origin, recognizing this pattern allows parents to explore alternative ways of expressing frustration and disappointment.

2. Silent Repression: Conversely, silent repression of anger can be equally detrimental. Acknowledging a tendency to internalize anger and avoid confrontation prompts parents to develop assertive communication skills.

Shaping a New Emotional Landscape

Breaking generational patterns is not just about cessation; it is about actively shaping a new emotional landscape within the family. This requires intentional efforts to foster emotional intelligence and resilience.

1. Open Communication: Establishing open communication channels is paramount. Creating an environment where family members feel comfortable expressing their

emotions without fear of judgment fosters healthier ways of addressing anger.

2. Teaching Emotional Regulation: Actively teaching children emotional regulation skills empowers them to navigate anger constructively. This includes providing tools such as deep breathing exercises, mindfulness techniques, and effective communication strategies.

Seeking Support and Guidance

Breaking generational patterns may necessitate seeking external support and guidance. Therapeutic interventions provide a safe space to explore the complexities of inherited patterns and develop strategies for transformative change.

1. Family Counseling: Family counseling offers a collaborative platform where generational patterns can be openly discussed and addressed. A therapist can guide the family in developing effective

communication skills and coping mechanisms.

2. Individual Therapy: Individual therapy provides parents with a personalized space for self-exploration. It allows them to delve into the roots of inherited patterns, fostering personal growth and empowering them to break free from detrimental cycles.

Cultivating Empathy and Understanding

Breaking generational patterns is not only about personal liberation but also about cultivating empathy and understanding within the family. It involves recognizing that each generation grapples with its unique challenges and offering compassion in the process of change.

1. Empathy for Past Generations: Acknowledging the challenges faced by past generations in expressing and managing anger cultivates empathy. Understanding that certain behaviors were learned in

response to specific circumstances fosters a compassionate perspective.

2. Creating a Culture of Understanding: Building a culture of understanding within the family involves encouraging open dialogue about generational influences. It creates an atmosphere where family members collaboratively work towards breaking detrimental patterns.

The Legacy of Emotional Mastery

Breaking generational patterns is a profound legacy—a gift that transcends individual experiences and shapes the emotional landscape for future generations. It is an investment in creating a family dynamic characterized by emotional intelligence, resilience, and a mastery of anger management.

1. Embracing Change as a Family Value: Making the commitment to break generational patterns becomes a shared

family value. Embracing change as a collective endeavor strengthens the resolve to prioritize emotional well-being.

2. Fostering Emotional Intelligence in Children: As parents actively work towards breaking generational patterns, they simultaneously foster emotional intelligence in their children. This equips the next generation with the tools to navigate emotions effectively and break free from inherited cycles.

Breaking generational patterns is a liberation—an intentional and transformative journey toward emotional mastery. It is a commitment to shaping a family environment that prioritizes understanding, resilience, and the conscious management of anger. By embarking on this journey, parents not only liberate themselves from the constraints of the past but also gift their children with the invaluable legacy of emotional well-being and mastery. The echoes of this liberation resonate through generations, creating a ripple effect of positive change within the family dynamic.

3.2 Stress and Parenting

In the intricate landscape of parental anger management, stress emerges as a formidable adversary. This chapter delves into the profound relationship between stress and parenting, offering insights and strategies for mastering emotions amid the challenges of raising children. By understanding the dynamics of stress and adopting effective coping mechanisms, parents can navigate the complex terrain of parenthood with resilience and emotional mastery.

The Interplay of Stress and Parenting

Parenting is a multifaceted journey marked by joy, fulfillment, and, inevitably, stress. The demands of raising children, coupled with external pressures, create a breeding ground for stress, which can significantly impact a parent's ability to manage anger effectively.

1. Daily Pressures: Juggling work, household responsibilities, and children's needs can create a daily pressure cooker. The accumulation of stressors, both big and small, contributes to heightened emotional responses, including anger.

2. Parental Expectations: Expectations placed on parents, whether societal or self-imposed, contribute to the stress load. Striving for perfection or succumbing to comparison can alleviate stress levels, influencing how parents navigate challenges and express emotions.

Recognizing Stress Triggers

To master anger management in the context of parenting, it is crucial to recognize the specific stress triggers that activate emotional responses. Identifying these triggers allows parents to intervene proactively and implement coping strategies.

1. Time Constraints: The perpetual race against time is a common stressor for parents. Recognizing the impact of time constraints on stress levels prompts a reassessment of priorities and time management strategies.

2. Sleep Deprivation: Lack of sleep is a potent stressor that amplifies emotional reactivity. Parents who recognize the connection between sleep and stress can prioritize adequate rest as a foundational aspect of anger management.

Coping Strategies for Parental Stress

Effectively managing stress is integral to anger management mastery. Adopting proactive coping strategies empowers parents to navigate challenges with a calm and collected demeanor.

1. Mindfulness and Relaxation Techniques: Incorporating mindfulness practices and relaxation techniques into daily routines fosters a grounded and present mindset. Techniques such as deep breathing, meditation, or yoga provide moments of respite amidst the chaos.

2. Establishing Support Systems: Building a support network is essential for stress management. Whether through friends, family, or support groups, having outlets for sharing concerns and seeking advice alleviates the emotional burden.

3. Setting Realistic Expectations: Managing stress involves setting realistic expectations for oneself. Recognizing that perfection is unattainable and embracing the ebb and flow of parenthood cultivates a more adaptable mindset.

Communicating Under Stress

Effective communication becomes paramount when stress levels rise. Navigating conversations with children and partners requires a mindful approach that considers the emotional climate created by stress.

1. Using "I" Statements: Expressing emotions through "I" statements fosters open communication without placing blame. This approach allows parents to share their feelings without escalating tension.

2. Active Listening: Stress can hinder active listening, leading to misunderstandings. Taking the time to listen attentively to children and partners enhances understanding and promotes a more supportive family dynamic.

Model Emotional Regulation

Parents serve as primary role models for their children. Modeling effective emotional regulation amid stress not only contributes to parental anger management but also equips children with invaluable skills for their own emotional well-being.

1. Expressing Emotions Positively: Demonstrating healthy ways to express and manage emotions sets a positive example. Parents who openly communicate about their feelings provide children with a blueprint for navigating their own emotional landscape.

2. Teaching Coping Strategies: Actively teaching children coping strategies for managing stress contributes to their emotional resilience. Whether through creative outlets, physical activity, or mindfulness, children can learn to navigate stress in constructive ways.

Seeking Professional Support

In cases where stress becomes overwhelming, seeking professional support is a proactive step toward maintaining emotional well-being. Therapists and counselors offer valuable guidance in developing coping strategies and addressing underlying stressors.

1. Individual Counseling: Individual counseling provides a confidential space for parents to explore the sources of stress and develop personalized coping mechanisms. Therapists can assist in reframing perspectives and building resilience.

2. Family Therapy: Family therapy offers a collaborative environment to address stressors that impact the entire family. It enhances communication skills, strengthens relationships, and fosters a supportive family dynamic.

Creating a Stress-Resilient Family Environment

Mastering anger management in the context of parenting involves creating a stress-resilient family environment. This requires a collective effort to prioritize emotional well-being and support each other through the inevitable challenges of parenthood.

1. Family Meetings: Regular family meetings provide an opportunity to discuss concerns, share feelings, and collaboratively problem-solve. Establishing an open forum for communication fosters a sense of unity in navigating stressors.

2. Celebrating Achievements: Acknowledging and celebrating achievements, no matter how small, contributes to a positive family atmosphere. Recognizing efforts and expressing gratitude cultivates a culture of support and resilience.

Navigating stress in the realm of parenting is an integral aspect of mastering anger management. By recognizing stress triggers, adopting coping strategies, and fostering effective communication, parents can create a family environment characterized by emotional intelligence, resilience, and a collective commitment to well-being. The journey toward emotional mastery amid stress is not a solitary endeavor but a shared commitment to nurturing a harmonious and emotionally resilient family dynamic.

3.2.1 Balancing Parenting Responsibilities

Parenting responsibilities, though rewarding, can create a delicate balance between joy and stress. This chapter delves into the intricate dance of balancing the myriad tasks of parenthood and the essential role this plays in mastering emotions, particularly anger. By understanding the challenges, adopting effective time-management strategies, and cultivating emotional intelligence, parents can navigate the complexities of parenting with grace and emotional mastery.

The Juggling Act of Parenting

Balancing parenting responsibilities involves juggling an array of tasks, from daily caregiving to managing household affairs and meeting professional commitments. The demands of parenthood can create a pressure cooker where emotions, including anger, may surface.

1. Time Constraints: The perpetual race against time is a common stressor for parents. Balancing work, childcare, and personal needs can lead to feelings of overwhelm, impacting emotional responses.

2. Unforeseen Challenges: Parenthood is rife with unforeseen challenges – from sudden illnesses to unexpected school projects. Navigating these surprises requires flexibility and adaptability, factors that influence emotional resilience.

Recognizing Stress Points

Identifying stress points within the realm of parenting responsibilities is essential for effective anger management. By recognizing triggers and acknowledging the sources of stress, parents can implement targeted strategies to maintain emotional equilibrium.

1. Overcommitment: Taking on too many responsibilities, whether at work or in the community, can lead to overcommitment. Recognizing the signs of overload allows parents to reassess priorities and set realistic expectations.

2. Lack of Personal Time: Depriving oneself of personal time and self-care exacerbates stress. Parents who recognize the importance of personal rejuvenation can establish boundaries and carve out moments for relaxation.

Time-Management Strategies

Effectively managing time is a cornerstone of balancing parenting responsibilities. Strategic time-management not only reduces stress but also creates space for intentional and mindful interactions with children.

1. Prioritizing Tasks: Identifying and prioritizing tasks based on urgency and importance allows parents to allocate time efficiently. This strategic approach minimizes the risk of feeling overwhelmed by an unmanageable workload.

2. Creating Routines: Establishing routines fosters predictability and stability for both parents and children. Routines provide a framework for managing responsibilities and reduce the likelihood of last-minute crises.

Cultivating Emotional Intelligence

Emotional intelligence plays a pivotal role in managing anger amid parenting responsibilities. By cultivating self-awareness and understanding the emotional needs of children, parents can respond to challenges with empathy and composure.

1. Self-Reflection Practices: Regular self-reflection allows parents to explore their emotional landscape. Journaling or mindfulness practices provide an outlet for processing emotions and gaining insights into personal triggers.

2. Empathetic Communication: Cultivating empathetic communication involves actively listening to children's needs and expressing emotions with sensitivity. This approach fosters mutual understanding and strengthens the parent-child bond.

Effective Communication with Co-Parents

For parents sharing responsibilities, effective communication is paramount. Coordinating tasks, discussing parenting strategies, and providing mutual support contribute to a harmonious and balanced parenting dynamic.

1. Scheduled Check-Ins: Regular check-ins with co-parents create opportunities to discuss schedules, address concerns, and share responsibilities. These meetings enhance communication and prevent misunderstandings.

2. Delegating Responsibilities: Delegating tasks and responsibilities ensures a fair distribution of the parenting load. Co-parents who collaborate in this way create a supportive partnership that minimizes stress.

The Role of Flexibility in Balancing Responsibilities

Flexibility is a crucial element in the delicate dance of balancing parenting responsibilities. Being adaptable to unexpected changes and embracing imperfections allows parents to navigate challenges with resilience and grace.

1. Embracing Imperfection: Accepting that perfection is unattainable liberates parents from unrealistic expectations. Embracing imperfections fosters a nurturing environment where mistakes are viewed as opportunities for growth.

2. Adjusting Expectations: Flexibility involves adjusting expectations based on the ebb and flow of family life. Parents who can adapt to changing circumstances cultivate a mindset that enhances emotional well-being.

Seeking Support and Outsourcing

Balancing parenting responsibilities does not mean going it alone. Seeking support from family, friends, or professional services can alleviate the burden, promoting emotional balance.

1. Family Support: Engaging with extended family for support, whether in childcare or household tasks, creates a sense of shared responsibility. Family support networks contribute to a more harmonious parenting experience.

2. Professional Assistance: Outsourcing tasks when possible, such as hiring help for specific household chores, eases the burden on parents. Professional assistance allows for more quality time with children and reduces stress.

Creating Moments of Connection

Amid the hustle and bustle of parenting responsibilities, creating moments of connection with children becomes paramount. These moments provide opportunities for bonding, fostering a positive emotional climate within the family.

1. Quality Time: Designating quality time for focused interaction strengthens the

parent-child relationship. Whether through shared activities or meaningful conversations, these moments contribute to emotional connection.

2.   Celebrating Achievements: Acknowledging and celebrating small achievements, both for parents and children, creates a positive atmosphere. This practice reinforces a sense of accomplishment and mutual appreciation.

Balancing parenting responsibilities is a dynamic and ongoing process that significantly influences emotional mastery, particularly in managing anger. By recognizing stress points, implementing effective time-management strategies, and cultivating emotional intelligence, parents can navigate the complexities of parenthood with resilience and grace. The journey toward emotional mastery within the context of balancing responsibilities is not a destination but an ongoing practice—a commitment to fostering a family environment characterized by understanding, connection, and a harmonious balance between parental duties and emotional well-being.

3.2.2 Managing External Stressors

Parenting, a rewarding and complex journey, often intersects with various external stressors. This chapter explores the crucial role of managing external stressors in the context of anger management for parents. By understanding the sources of stress, developing coping strategies, and fostering resilience, parents can master their emotions and create a more harmonious family environment.

The Impact of External Stressors on Parenting

External stressors, ranging from financial pressures to societal expectations, can significantly influence a parent's emotional well-being. Recognizing the potential impact of these stressors is the first step toward effective anger management.

1. Financial Strain: Financial challenges can evoke feelings of frustration and helplessness. Parents grappling with economic stress may find it challenging to separate these concerns from their parenting responsibilities.

2. Work-Parenting Balance: Juggling work and parenting responsibilities is a common stressor. The demands of the workplace and the desire to be present for children can create a delicate balance that, if not managed, may lead to heightened emotions.

Identifying Sources of External Stress

Understanding specific sources of external stress allows parents to tailor their anger management strategies. Identification enables proactive measures to address stressors before they escalate.

1. Parental Comparison: The pervasive culture of parental comparison, fueled by social media and societal expectations, can induce stress. Acknowledging the impact of comparison on emotions is essential for effective anger management.

2. Societal Expectations: Societal pressures and expectations regarding parenting styles and achievements can contribute to stress. Parental self-awareness and the ability to set realistic expectations are vital in managing these external influences.

Coping Strategies for External Stressors

Developing effective coping strategies is crucial in mastering emotions in the face of external stressors. By incorporating proactive measures, parents can build resilience and navigate challenges with composure.

1. Mindfulness Practices: Engaging in mindfulness practices, such as meditation or

mindful breathing, fosters a grounded and present mindset. These practices offer a reprieve from external stressors, allowing parents to approach challenges with clarity.

2. Establishing Boundaries: Creating clear boundaries between work and personal life helps manage the stress of balancing professional and parenting responsibilities. Establishing designated times for work and family contributes to a more balanced lifestyle.

Communication Strategies for Coping

Effective communication becomes a crucial tool in managing external stressors. Open dialogue with family members and co-parents fosters a supportive environment and prevents emotions from escalating.

1. Family Meetings: Regular family meetings provide a platform for discussing external stressors and collaboratively finding solutions. Transparent communication

ensures that everyone is on the same page, reducing potential conflicts.

2. Co-Parenting Communication: Coordinating with co-parents through open and honest communication is paramount. Discussing external stressors and sharing responsibilities prevents misunderstandings and fosters a unified approach to parenting.

Building Resilience in the Face of Challenges

Resilience is a key attribute in mastering emotions amid external stressors. Building resilience involves developing a mindset that views challenges as opportunities for growth rather than insurmountable obstacles.

1. Learning from Adversity: Viewing challenges as opportunities for learning and growth reframes the narrative around stressors. Embracing adversity as part of the

parenting journey promotes emotional resilience.

2. Seeking Support: Recognizing when external stressors become overwhelming and seeking support is a sign of resilience. Whether through friends, family, or professional assistance, reaching out contributes to emotional well-being.

Creating a Supportive Network

A robust support network is instrumental in navigating external stressors. Cultivating connections with friends, family, and community resources provides a safety net during challenging times.

1. Friendship Circles: Building friendships with other parents creates a sense of camaraderie. Sharing experiences and providing mutual support establishes a valuable network for navigating external stressors.

2. Community Involvement: Engaging with community resources, such as parenting groups or local organizations, expands the support network. Community involvement offers diverse perspectives and assistance in managing external challenges.

Maintaining Perspective and Self-Reflection

Maintaining perspective in the face of external stressors is essential for emotional mastery. Regular self-reflection allows parents to assess their emotional responses and adjust their mindset accordingly.

1. Perspective Shift: Adopting a broader perspective on external stressors helps parents see the bigger picture. Recognizing that challenges are temporary and surmountable fosters a resilient mindset.

2. Journaling and Reflection: Journaling and regular self-reflection provide a platform for processing emotions. By documenting

thoughts and feelings, parents gain insight into their emotional responses and can identify patterns.

Seeking Professional Guidance

In instances where external stressors become overwhelming, seeking professional guidance is a proactive step. Therapists and counselors offer valuable insights and coping strategies to manage emotions effectively.

1. Individual Therapy: Individual therapy provides a confidential space for parents to explore the emotional impact of external stressors. Therapists can assist in developing personalized coping mechanisms and fostering emotional resilience.

2. Family Counseling: Family counseling offers a collaborative environment to address stressors affecting the entire family. It enhances communication skills and

provides strategies for managing external challenges collectively.

Cultivating a Positive Parenting Mindset

Cultivating a positive parenting mindset involves consciously shaping thoughts and attitudes in response to external stressors. This proactive approach contributes to emotional mastery and a more harmonious family environment.

1. Gratitude Practices: Incorporating gratitude practices into daily routines shifts the focus from stressors to positive aspects of parenting. Acknowledging and appreciating moments of joy fosters a more optimistic mindset.

2. Affirmations and Positive Self-Talk: Utilizing affirmations and positive self-talk counteracts negative thoughts arising from external stressors. Encouraging oneself with affirming statements promotes emotional resilience.

Mastering emotions in the face of external stressors is a dynamic and ongoing journey. By understanding sources of stress, implementing effective coping strategies, and fostering resilience, parents can navigate the complexities of parenting with emotional mastery. The ability to manage anger in the context of external stressors not only promotes individual well-being but also contributes to a positive and nurturing family environment. The journey is a testament to the resilience and strength of parents who, in navigating external challenges, ultimately create a legacy of emotional mastery for generations to come.

Chapter 4: The Power of Self-Awareness

4.1 Cultivating Self-Awareness

In the labyrinth of parenthood, cultivating self-awareness emerges as the keystone for mastering emotions, especially in the face of anger. This chapter delves into the profound significance of self-awareness for parents, exploring its transformative power in understanding and regulating emotions. By embarking on a journey of self-discovery, parents can navigate the complexities of anger management with insight, resilience, and a commitment to emotional mastery.

The Essence of Self-Awareness in Parenting

Self-awareness, the ability to recognize and understand one's thoughts, emotions, and behaviors, is a powerful tool for emotional regulation. In the context of parenting, cultivating self-awareness is akin to holding a mirror to one's internal landscape, shedding light on the intricate interplay of emotions that can lead to anger.

1. Recognizing Triggers: Self-awareness enables parents to identify specific triggers that activate anger. Whether it's fatigue, stress, or unmet expectations, understanding these triggers provides a foundation for effective anger management.

2. Understanding Emotional Responses: Delving into the nuances of emotional responses allows parents to decipher the underlying feelings beneath anger. This awareness empowers parents to address root emotions rather than solely reacting to surface-level anger.

The Journey of Self-Discovery

Cultivating self-awareness is a journey of self-discovery, involving introspection, reflection, and a willingness to explore the depths of one's emotional landscape. It is an ongoing process that unfolds over time, offering profound insights into the dynamics of parenthood and emotional regulation.

1. Journaling as a Reflective Practice: Maintaining a journal becomes a valuable tool for self-reflection. By documenting thoughts, emotions, and reactions, parents create a tangible record that facilitates deeper understanding and pattern recognition.

2. Mindfulness Practices: Incorporating mindfulness into daily routines enhances self-awareness. Mindful practices, such as meditation or mindful breathing, anchor parents in the present moment, fostering an acute awareness of their emotional state.

Unraveling the Roots of Anger

Self-awareness invites parents to unravel the roots of their anger, exploring the origins and patterns that influence emotional responses. This exploration is instrumental in breaking the cycle of reactive anger and fostering intentional, measured responses.

1. Exploring Childhood Influences: Childhood experiences shape emotional responses in adulthood. Self-awareness involves examining the influences of one's upbringing, identifying learned patterns, and addressing any unresolved emotions from the past.

2. Examining Personal Triggers: Identifying personal triggers that activate anger is a crucial aspect of self-awareness. Whether it's a specific behavior, circumstance, or internal thought, recognizing these triggers empowers parents to respond more consciously.

The Role of Emotional Intelligence

Self-awareness is intertwined with emotional intelligence, a set of skills that encompasses recognizing, understanding, and managing one's own emotions, as well as empathizing with the emotions of others. In the context of anger management, emotional intelligence provides a roadmap for navigating the complex terrain of parental emotions.

1. Recognizing Emotional Cues: Emotional intelligence involves recognizing subtle cues that precede the escalation of anger. This heightened awareness allows parents to intervene at an early stage, preventing the intensification of emotional reactions.

2. Empathy Toward Children's Emotions: Cultivating empathy toward children's emotions is a pivotal aspect of emotional intelligence. Understanding the perspectives and feelings of children creates a more compassionate approach to parenting and anger management.

Integrating Self-Awareness into Parenting Practices

The true essence of self-awareness lies in its integration into everyday parenting practices. It is not a theoretical concept but a lived experience that shapes interactions, responses, and the overall emotional climate within the family.

1. Pause and Reflect: Incorporating moments of pause and reflection into daily routines allows parents to check in with their emotional state. A brief pause before reacting creates space for conscious choices rather than impulsive responses.

2. Communication Through "I" Statements: Effective communication is rooted in self-awareness. Using "I" statements to express feelings, thoughts, and needs fosters open dialogue and prevents the escalation of anger through blame.

The Challenge of Acceptance

Self-awareness also involves the challenge of self-acceptance—a willingness to embrace the full spectrum of emotions without judgment. This acceptance creates a foundation for authentic expression and a healthier relationship with anger.

1. Embracing Imperfection: Acknowledging that perfection is unattainable liberates parents from self-imposed expectations. Embracing imperfection fosters self-compassion and resilience in the face of challenges.

2. Learning from Mistakes: Self-awareness includes the capacity to learn from mistakes. Instead of dwelling on perceived failures, parents who view mistakes as opportunities for growth cultivate a positive and evolving mindset.

Seeking External Support

In the journey of cultivating self-awareness, seeking external support can provide additional perspectives and insights. Whether through conversations with trusted friends, participation in support groups, or professional counseling, external support enhances the self-awareness process.

1. Therapeutic Guidance: Individual or family therapy offers a structured and supportive environment for exploring self-awareness. Therapists provide guidance, feedback, and tools for enhancing emotional regulation within the family dynamic.

2. Peer Support: Engaging with other parents in similar journeys fosters a sense of community. Peer support provides opportunities for shared experiences, insights, and encouragement in the pursuit of self-awareness.

A Legacy of Emotional Mastery

Cultivating self-awareness is not only a personal endeavor but a legacy that shapes the emotional landscape of the entire family. As parents embark on this journey of self-discovery, they lay the groundwork for a legacy of emotional mastery—an invaluable gift passed on to future generations.

1. Role Modeling Emotional Regulation: Parents who actively cultivate self-awareness serve as powerful role models for their children. Children observe and internalize the importance of self-reflection, emotional understanding, and intentional responses.

2. Creating a Nurturing Family Environment: A family environment rooted in self-awareness is characterized by open communication, empathy, and a shared commitment to emotional well-being. This nurturing environment becomes a sanctuary

for growth, understanding, and emotional mastery.

In the tapestry of parenthood, self-awareness is the thread that weaves together emotional mastery and effective anger management. By embarking on the journey of self-discovery, parents unlock the transformative power of understanding and regulating their emotions. The commitment to self-awareness is a commitment to creating a family environment characterized by empathy, resilience, and a shared journey toward emotional mastery—a legacy that reverberates through the generations.

4.1.1 Mindfulness Practices

In the intricate dance of parenthood, where emotions ebb and flow, mindfulness emerges as a powerful ally in the pursuit of anger management mastery. This chapter delves into the transformative potential of mindfulness practices, exploring how they can empower parents to be the masters of their emotions, fostering resilience, and creating a harmonious family dynamic.

The Essence of Mindfulness in Parenting

Mindfulness, rooted in ancient contemplative traditions, is the practice of being fully present in the current moment without judgment. In the context of parenting, mindfulness becomes a compass that guides parents through the challenges, frustrations, and joys, offering a sanctuary of calm amidst the whirlwind of emotions.

1. Present-Moment Awareness: Mindfulness invites parents to anchor themselves in the present moment, free from the entanglements of past regrets or future anxieties. This awareness creates a mental space for intentional responses rather than reactive emotions.

2. Non-Judgmental Observation: The non-judgmental aspect of mindfulness encourages parents to observe their thoughts

and emotions without attaching value judgments. This detached observation fosters self-acceptance and reduces the likelihood of being swept away by intense emotions.

Incorporating Mindfulness into Daily Life

Mindfulness is not reserved for secluded meditation sessions; it can be seamlessly integrated into daily life. By infusing mindful practices into routine activities, parents can cultivate a sustained state of awareness and emotional regulation.

1. Mindful Breathing: Conscious attention to the breath is a fundamental mindfulness practice. Parents can incorporate mindful breathing during routine tasks, such as preparing meals or commuting, grounding themselves in the rhythm of inhalation and exhalation.

2. Mindful Eating: Turning mealtimes into mindful experiences allows parents to savor

each bite, engaging their senses fully. This practice not only nurtures physical well-being but also cultivates a mindful approach to daily activities.

Mindfulness in the Midst of Chaos

Parenthood often presents moments of chaos and unpredictability. Mindfulness equips parents with the tools to navigate these challenges with composure and intentional responses, preventing the escalation of anger.

1. Mindful Responses to Tantrums: When faced with a child's tantrum, a mindful parent takes a moment to breathe, observes their own emotional reactions, and responds with patience and understanding. This intentional response de-escalates the situation and models emotional regulation for the child.

2. Cultivating Patience: Mindfulness practices, such as mindful walking or body

scans, nurture patience. As parents cultivate the ability to embrace the present moment, impatience gives way to a more grounded and composed demeanor.

Mindfulness-Based Stress Reduction (MBSR)

Mindfulness-Based Stress Reduction (MBSR), developed by Dr. Jon Kabat-Zinn, is a structured program that incorporates mindfulness meditation to alleviate stress. For parents juggling multiple responsibilities, MBSR can be a transformative tool for managing stress and anger.

1. Mindful Body Scan: The body scan is a core component of MBSR, involving a focused awareness of each part of the body. Parents can engage in a brief body scan to release tension and cultivate a heightened awareness of physical sensations.

2. Mindful Meditation Sessions: Dedicated sessions of mindful meditation, even if brief, offer parents a respite from the demands of daily life. These sessions can be tailored to fit into busy schedules, providing a rejuvenating pause for emotional well-being.

Emotional Regulation Through Mindfulness

One of the profound benefits of mindfulness is its capacity to enhance emotional regulation. By fostering awareness of emotions and creating a mental space for intentional responses, mindfulness becomes a cornerstone for effective anger management.

1. Observing Emotions Non-Judgmentally: Mindfulness encourages parents to observe their emotions without judgment. When anger arises, a mindful parent acknowledges it without condemnation, allowing for a more conscious and measured response.

2. Mindful Check-Ins: Integrating mindful check-ins into daily routines involves pausing to assess one's emotional state. This brief moment of self-reflection empowers parents to recognize potential triggers and address them before emotions escalate.

Mindful Parenting and Connection

Mindful parenting is not only about individual well-being but also about fostering a deeper connection with children. By being fully present and attuned to the needs of their children, parents create a nurturing environment rooted in understanding and empathy.

1. Mindful Listening: Engaging in mindful listening involves giving full attention to what children express without immediate judgment or reaction. This practice fosters open communication and strengthens the parent-child bond.

2. Quality Time with Mindful Presence: Quality time becomes enriched when parents bring mindful presence to shared activities. Whether playing, reading, or engaging in conversations, the depth of connection deepens when both parent and child are fully present.

Mindfulness for Parental Well-Being

Parental well-being is intricately tied to the practice of mindfulness. By prioritizing self-care and emotional regulation, parents can create a sustainable foundation for navigating the challenges of parenthood.

1. Mindful Self-Compassion: Mindfulness extends to self-compassion, allowing parents to treat themselves with the same kindness and understanding they offer their children. Embracing self-compassion fosters emotional resilience and prevents self-criticism.

2. Mindful Movement Practices: Incorporating mindful movement practices, such as yoga or tai chi, into the routine promotes physical well-being and cultivates a sense of calm. These practices serve as a holistic approach to emotional and physical health.

Mindfulness and the Ripple Effect

The transformative power of mindfulness extends beyond individual well-being to influence the entire family dynamic. The ripple effect of mindfulness creates a harmonious atmosphere characterized by understanding, patience, and shared moments of presence.

1. Family Mindfulness Practices: Introducing simple mindfulness practices to the entire family, such as mindful walks or gratitude exercises, creates a collective commitment to emotional well-being. These shared practices foster a sense of unity and connection.

2. Teaching Children Mindfulness: Children can benefit from mindfulness practices tailored to their age. Teaching them simple techniques, like mindful breathing or guided imagery, equips them with valuable tools for emotional regulation.

In the kaleidoscope of parenthood, mindfulness emerges as a guiding light—a transformative practice that empowers parents to be the masters of their emotions. By cultivating present-moment awareness, integrating mindfulness into daily life, and embracing the ripple effect on the family dynamic, parents embark on a mindful journey toward emotional mastery. The commitment to mindfulness becomes a profound gift—a legacy that fosters resilience, connection, and a harmonious family environment for generations to come.

4.1.2 Journaling for Reflection

In the intricate tapestry of parenthood, where emotions ebb and flow like a tempestuous river, journaling emerges as a potent vessel for navigating the currents of anger. This chapter delves into the transformative potential of journaling for parents, exploring how this reflective practice can be a compass, guiding them towards emotional mastery, resilience, and a deeper understanding of their own parenting journey.

The Art of Journaling in Parenting

Journaling is more than ink on paper; it is a dynamic process of self-exploration and reflection. In the realm of parenting, it becomes a confidante, a space where the unfiltered nuances of emotions can be laid bare, and where the journey of anger management can be chronicled with honesty and vulnerability.

1. Private Dialogues on Paper: Journaling provides a safe haven for private dialogues

on paper. Parents can pour their thoughts, frustrations, and triumphs onto the pages, creating a tangible narrative of their emotional landscape.

2. Tracking Patterns and Triggers: Through consistent journaling, parents can track patterns and identify triggers that give rise to anger. This process of self-awareness lays the groundwork for targeted anger management strategies and interventions.

Journaling as a Reflective Practice

Reflective journaling is a deliberate practice that involves exploring thoughts and emotions with a discerning eye. In the context of anger management, it becomes a tool for dissecting the intricate threads of frustration, uncovering the root causes, and devising strategies for a measured response.

1. Daily Check-Ins: A daily check-in through journaling offers parents the opportunity to reflect on the highs and lows

of the day. It becomes a ritual of self-awareness, a moment to acknowledge emotions, and a chance to celebrate small victories.

2. Unraveling Anger Episodes: When anger flares, journaling serves as a post-mortem analysis of the episode. Parents can delve into the circumstances, their emotional state, and the triggers that led to anger. This reflective exploration lays the foundation for proactive measures.

The Emotional Catharsis of Journaling

Anger, when left unexpressed or unexamined, can fester like a storm cloud. Journaling becomes a form of emotional catharsis, allowing parents to release pent-up feelings, grapple with the intensity of emotions, and pave the way for a calmer internal landscape.

1. Expressive Writing: The act of writing itself becomes a form of expression.

Through expressive writing, parents can articulate their feelings with raw honesty, unburdening themselves of the weight of unspoken emotions.

2. Acknowledging Frustrations: Journaling provides a platform to acknowledge frustrations without judgment. By giving voice to the challenges and irritations, parents validate their own experiences and create space for emotional healing.

Setting Journaling Intentions

Intentionality transforms journaling from a mere record-keeping activity into a purposeful practice. By setting intentions for their journaling journey, parents can align this reflective process with specific goals related to anger management.

1. Intentions for Emotional Regulation: Journaling with the intention of enhancing emotional regulation involves exploring techniques and strategies that promote

calmness. This may include jotting down coping mechanisms or affirmations that resonate with the individual.

2. Goals for Positive Parenting: For parents aiming to foster positive parenting practices, journaling becomes a canvas for outlining specific goals. Whether it's cultivating patience, active listening, or empathy, journaling serves as a roadmap for intentional parenting.

Journaling Techniques for Anger Management

The spectrum of journaling techniques is vast, offering diverse approaches for exploring emotions and cultivating self-awareness. Tailoring journaling practices to suit individual preferences and needs enhances the effectiveness of this reflective tool.

1. Freewriting: Freewriting involves letting thoughts flow without inhibition. Parents

can use this technique to unload the contents of their mind onto paper, uncovering insights and patterns that may be hidden beneath the surface.

2. Prompt-Based Journaling: Using prompts adds structure to journaling. Parents can explore specific prompts related to anger management, such as "Today's triggers," or "Strategies for responding calmly," guiding their reflections in a focused direction.

Journaling Through Positive Reinforcement

While journaling is a powerful tool for exploring challenges, it can also be a platform for reinforcing positive aspects of parenting. Acknowledging successes, expressing gratitude, and capturing moments of joy contribute to a balanced and uplifting narrative.

1. Gratitude Journaling: Gratitude journaling involves noting down moments of gratitude and positive experiences. This practice shifts

the focus from challenges to blessings, fostering a mindset of appreciation and resilience.

2. Celebrating Milestones: Journaling becomes a chronicle of growth and achievements. By celebrating milestones, no matter how small, parents cultivate a sense of accomplishment and resilience, counterbalancing the inevitable challenges of parenthood.

The Long-Term Benefits of Journaling

The impact of journaling extends beyond immediate emotional relief; it lays the groundwork for sustained emotional well-being and growth. As parents embark on a consistent journaling practice, the benefits ripple through various dimensions of their lives.

1. Building Emotional Resilience: Journaling contributes to emotional resilience by providing an outlet for

processing challenges. The act of reflection and intentionality in responding to difficulties fosters a robust emotional foundation.

2. Cultivating a Growth Mindset: Over time, journaling becomes a testament to personal growth. Parents witness the evolution of their responses to anger, the acquisition of new coping strategies, and the development of a growth mindset that embraces challenges as opportunities for learning.

Seeking Support Through Journaling

Journaling can be a solitary endeavor, but it can also be a bridge to seeking external support. Sharing journal entries with a trusted friend, family member, or therapist provides an additional layer of insight and encouragement.

1. Therapeutic Journaling: Therapeutic journaling involves working with a therapist who guides the reflective process. This collaborative approach enhances the depth

of exploration and provides targeted strategies for anger management.

2. Sharing with a Support Network: Opening up journal entries for discussion within a support network creates opportunities for empathy and understanding. Fellow parents or friends can offer insights and perspectives that contribute to a richer understanding of one's emotions.

In the symphony of parenthood, where emotions compose the melodies, journaling becomes a compass guiding parents through the complex landscape of anger management. By embracing this reflective practice, parents embark on a journey of self-discovery, resilience, and intentional responses. Journaling is not merely a record; it is a dynamic process that transforms the act of parenting into a narrative of growth, understanding, and emotional mastery—a legacy that reverberates through the pages and the hearts of generations to come.

4.2 Recognizing Emotional Triggers in Real Time

In the intricate dance of parenthood, recognizing emotional triggers in real-time is akin to navigating the turbulent currents with precision. This chapter explores the profound importance of identifying triggers as they emerge, offering parents a roadmap for anger management mastery and the ability to be the architects of their emotional responses.

The Dynamics of Emotional Triggers

Emotional triggers are catalysts that propel individuals from a state of equilibrium to heightened emotional arousal. In the context of parenting, recognizing these triggers in real-time is a pivotal skill that empowers parents to respond with intentionality rather than succumbing to reactive emotions.

1. Definition of Triggers: Triggers can be external events, specific behaviors, or internal thoughts that evoke strong emotional responses. Recognizing these triggers is fundamental to unraveling the complex web of emotions that parents may experience.

2. Impact on Parental Responses: Emotional triggers have a direct impact on how parents respond to situations. Whether it's a challenging behavior from a child, a stressful situation, or a reminder of past experiences, triggers shape the emotional terrain of parenting.

The Significance of Real-Time Recognition

Identifying emotional triggers in the heat of the moment is a game-changer for effective anger management. Real-time recognition provides parents with the opportunity to pause, assess, and choose intentional responses, disrupting the automatic cycle of reactive behavior.

1. Preventing Escalation: Real-time recognition serves as a preventive measure against the escalation of anger. By identifying triggers in the early stages, parents can intervene before emotions intensify, fostering a more measured and composed response.

2. Enhancing Self-Awareness: Real-time recognition contributes to heightened self-awareness. Parents who can identify triggers in the moment gain insights into their emotional landscape, fostering a deeper understanding of the root causes of anger.

Types of Emotional Triggers in Parenthood

Emotional triggers in the realm of parenting are diverse and multifaceted. Recognizing these triggers requires a nuanced understanding of individual sensitivities, past experiences, and the unique dynamics of parent-child relationships.

1. Unmet Expectations: When expectations regarding children's behavior or outcomes are unmet, frustration can ensue. Real-time recognition allows parents to adjust expectations in the moment and respond with flexibility.

2. Feeling Overwhelmed: The demands of parenthood can lead to feelings of overwhelm. Recognizing this emotional trigger enables parents to implement self-care strategies in real-time, mitigating stress and preventing the buildup of frustration.

3. Challenging Behaviors: Specific behaviors displayed by children, such as defiance or disobedience, can serve as triggers. Real-time recognition allows parents to address these behaviors with patience and understanding, rather than reacting impulsively.

Strategies for Real-Time Recognition

Developing the ability to recognize emotional triggers in real-time is a skill that can be honed through intentional practices. These strategies empower parents to be proactive in their approach to anger management.

1. Mindful Awareness: Cultivating mindfulness involves being fully present in the moment. In real-time, parents can practice mindful awareness by observing their thoughts, emotions, and physical sensations without judgment.

2. Breathing Techniques: Employing conscious breathing techniques provides a practical tool for real-time recognition. Taking slow, deep breaths creates a pause, allowing parents to assess their emotional state and choose a measured response.

3. Self-Reflective Pause: Creating a habit of taking a self-reflective pause in challenging situations is a powerful strategy. This pause, even if brief, serves as a moment to identify emerging triggers and consciously choose a response.

Cultivating Real-Time Response Strategies

Once emotional triggers are recognized, the next step is to cultivate effective strategies for real-time response. These strategies empower parents to navigate challenges with composure and foster a positive emotional climate within the family.

1. Active Listening: In the midst of a potential trigger, active listening becomes a powerful response strategy. Real-time recognition allows parents to attune themselves to their child's perspective, fostering empathy and connection.

2. Verbalizing Emotions: Expressing emotions verbally in real-time serves a dual purpose. It allows parents to acknowledge their own feelings and model emotional expression for their children. This transparent communication contributes to a climate of open dialogue.

The Role of Communication in Real-Time Recognition

Communication plays a pivotal role in recognizing emotional triggers in real-time. Effective communication, both with oneself and with children, becomes a bridge to understanding, empathy, and the cultivation of a positive emotional environment.

1. Internal Dialogue: Maintaining an internal dialogue in real-time involves consciously narrating one's thoughts and emotions. This self-talk serves as a tool for processing feelings and making intentional choices in response to triggers.

2. Expressing Needs: Real-time recognition enables parents to express their needs assertively and constructively. Communicating needs fosters a collaborative approach, allowing for resolution and preventing the escalation of anger.

Building Resilience Through Real-Time Recognition

Real-time recognition of emotional triggers is not only a strategy for managing anger; it is a cornerstone for building emotional resilience. By navigating challenges with precision and intentionality, parents cultivate a resilient mindset that withstands the complexities of parenthood.

1. Learning from Each Experience: Real-time recognition serves as an ongoing learning process. Each instance becomes an opportunity for growth, self-discovery, and the refinement of response strategies.

2. Embracing Imperfection: Recognizing triggers in real-time involves embracing the imperfections of the parenting journey. Parents who acknowledge their vulnerabilities and navigate challenges with self-compassion foster resilience in the face of adversity.

Seeking Professional Guidance for Real-Time Recognition

For parents facing persistent challenges in recognizing emotional triggers, seeking professional guidance can provide valuable insights and support. Therapists or counselors can offer tailored strategies and facilitate a deeper exploration of individual triggers.

1. Therapeutic Intervention: Therapeutic interventions focus on the real-time recognition of triggers within the therapeutic setting. Therapists guide parents through the exploration of triggers, offering tools and strategies for effective anger management.

2. Skill-Building Workshops:
Participating in skill-building workshops enhances the capacity for real-time recognition. These workshops provide practical techniques, scenarios for practice, and a supportive environment for learning and growth.

In the intricate landscape of parenthood, recognizing emotional triggers in real-time is an art—a skill that transforms the chaotic into the manageable. By honing this skill, parents navigate the twists and turns of the emotional terrain with precision, responding to challenges with intentionality and fostering a positive family dynamic. Real-time recognition becomes the compass that guides parents toward emotional mastery, resilience, and the ability to be the architects of their parenting journey—creating a legacy of understanding, connection, and emotional well-being for generations to come.

4.2.1 The Role of Mindfulness in Anger Management

In the intricate tapestry of parenthood, where emotions ebb and flow like a river, mindfulness emerges as a powerful beacon illuminating the path to anger management mastery. This chapter delves into the profound role of mindfulness, exploring how it empowers parents to be the masters of their emotions, fostering resilience, and creating a harmonious family dynamic.

Understanding Mindfulness in the Parenting Context

Mindfulness, rooted in ancient contemplative traditions, is the practice of being fully present in the current moment without judgment. In the context of parenting, it becomes a transformative lens through which parents can navigate the challenges of anger management.

1. Present-Moment Awareness: Mindfulness invites parents to anchor themselves in the present moment. Amidst the chaos of parenting, this awareness provides a sanctuary, a mental space where intentional responses can blossom.

2. Non-Judgmental Observation: A core tenet of mindfulness is the non-judgmental observation of thoughts and emotions. For parents, this means observing their own reactions without attaching value judgments, fostering self-acceptance and reducing the impact of self-criticism.

The Power of Mindfulness in Real-Time Anger Management

Mindfulness isn't a theoretical concept; it's a practice that unfolds in real-time, especially in the crucible of anger management. Here's how mindfulness functions as a powerful tool in those critical moments.

1. Interrupting Automatic Responses: Mindfulness creates a pause between stimulus and response. In the face of a triggering event, parents can leverage this pause to interrupt automatic reactions, providing the space for a more thoughtful and measured response.

2. Cultivating Emotional Regulation: The essence of mindfulness lies in cultivating emotional regulation. By fostering an awareness of emotions as they arise, parents can navigate the turbulence of anger with greater poise, preventing its escalation.

Mindfulness in Daily Life

The beauty of mindfulness lies in its integration into the fabric of daily life. It's not reserved for meditation sessions alone; it permeates routine activities, transforming them into opportunities for heightened awareness.

1. Mindful Breathing: Simple yet profound, mindful breathing involves paying attention to each breath. Parents can infuse mindful breathing into daily routines, grounding themselves in the rhythm of inhalation and exhalation, especially in moments of stress.

2. Mindful Presence in Routine Tasks: Washing dishes, playing with children, or cooking a meal can become occasions for mindful presence. By immersing themselves fully in these activities, parents cultivate an attitude of awareness and intentionality.

Mindfulness Amidst the Storm of Parenthood

Parenthood, at times, resembles a storm where emotions surge unpredictably. Mindfulness equips parents with tools to weather the storm, fostering calmness and intentional responses even in the face of chaos.

1. Mindful Responses to Tantrums: When confronted with a child's tantrum, mindfulness allows parents to step back, observe their own emotional reactions, and respond with patience and understanding. This intentional response not only de-escalates the situation but also models emotional regulation.

2. Cultivating Patience Through Mindfulness: Mindfulness practices, such as mindful walking or body scans, nurture patience. In cultivating the ability to embrace the present moment, parents find that impatience gradually gives way to a more composed demeanor.

Mindfulness-Based Stress Reduction (MBSR)

Developed by Dr. Jon Kabat-Zinn, Mindfulness-Based Stress Reduction

(MBSR) is a structured program that incorporates mindfulness meditation to alleviate stress. For parents juggling myriad responsibilities, MBSR offers a transformative approach to anger management.

1. Mindful Body Scan: Central to MBSR is the mindful body scan, a practice involving focused attention on each part of the body. Parents can engage in a brief body scan to release tension and cultivate heightened awareness of physical sensations.

2. Mindful Meditation Sessions: Incorporating dedicated sessions of mindful meditation into daily routines provides a reprieve from the demands of parenting. These sessions need not be lengthy; even brief moments of focused attention contribute to emotional well-being.

Emotional Intelligence Through Mindfulness

Mindfulness and emotional intelligence are intertwined. Emotional intelligence involves recognizing, understanding, and managing one's own emotions, as well as empathizing with the emotions of others. In the context of anger management, mindfulness becomes a cornerstone for enhancing emotional intelligence.

1. Recognizing Emotional Cues: Mindfulness sharpens the ability to recognize subtle emotional cues that precede anger. This heightened awareness empowers parents to intervene at an early stage, preventing the escalation of emotional reactions.

2. Empathy Toward Children's Emotions: Cultivating empathy toward children's emotions is a pivotal aspect of emotional intelligence. By understanding their perspectives and feelings, parents foster a more compassionate approach to parenting and anger management.

Mindful Parenting Practices

Mindfulness extends beyond individual well-being to influence parenting practices. By infusing mindfulness into the parent-child dynamic, parents create an environment characterized by understanding, patience, and open communication.

1. Mindful Listening: Engaging in mindful listening involves giving full attention to what children express without immediate judgment or reaction. This practice fosters open communication and strengthens the parent-child bond.

2. Quality Time with Mindful Presence: Shared activities become enriched when parents bring mindful presence to the moment. Whether playing, reading, or conversing, the depth of connection deepens when both parent and child are fully engaged.

Mindfulness for Personal Well-Being

Mindfulness is not only a tool for managing anger; it is a catalyst for personal well-being. By prioritizing self-care and emotional regulation, parents create a sustainable foundation for navigating the challenges of parenthood.

1. Mindful Self-Compassion: Mindfulness extends to self-compassion, allowing parents to treat themselves with the same kindness and understanding they offer their children. Embracing self-compassion fosters emotional resilience and prevents self-criticism.

2. Mindful Movement Practices: Incorporating mindful movement practices, such as yoga or tai chi, into the routine promotes physical well-being and cultivates a sense of calm. These practices serve as a holistic approach to emotional and physical health.

Mindfulness and the Ripple Effect

The transformative power of mindfulness extends beyond individual well-being to influence the entire family dynamic. The ripple effect of mindfulness creates a harmonious atmosphere characterized by understanding, patience, and shared moments of presence.

1. Family Mindfulness Practices: Introducing simple mindfulness practices to the entire family, such as mindful walks or gratitude exercises, creates a collective commitment to emotional well-being. These shared practices foster a sense of unity and connection.

2. Teaching Children Mindfulness: Children can benefit from mindfulness practices tailored to their age. Teaching them simple techniques, like mindful breathing or guided imagery, equips them with valuable tools for emotional regulation.

In the mosaic of parenthood, mindfulness emerges as a guiding light—a transformative practice that empowers parents to be the masters of their emotions. By cultivating present-moment awareness, integrating mindfulness into daily life, and embracing the ripple effect on the family dynamic, parents embark on a mindful journey toward emotional mastery. The commitment to mindfulness becomes a profound gift—a legacy that reverberates through the generations, fostering resilience, connection, and a harmonious family environment for years to come.

Chapter 5: Strategies for Anger Management

5.1 Developing Healthy Coping Mechanisms

In the labyrinth of parenthood, where emotions weave a complex tapestry, the development of healthy coping mechanisms is akin to forging a resilient shield against the challenges that anger may present. This chapter delves into the transformative journey of cultivating coping strategies, empowering parents to be the architects of their emotional responses and fostering a harmonious family dynamic.

The Crucial Role of Coping Mechanisms

Coping mechanisms are the strategies individuals employ to navigate stress, challenges, and intense emotions. In the context of parenting, developing healthy coping mechanisms is not just a practical necessity but a profound investment in emotional well-being.

1. Definition of Coping Mechanisms: Coping mechanisms encompass a range of behaviors, thoughts, and actions that individuals use to manage and navigate difficult situations. These mechanisms can be adaptive and constructive or maladaptive and potentially harmful.

2. Impact on Parental Well-Being: The quality of coping mechanisms directly influences parental well-being. Effective coping strategies contribute to emotional resilience, allowing parents to weather the storms of parenthood with grace and intentionality.

Identifying Unhealthy Coping Mechanisms

Before delving into the development of healthy coping mechanisms, it's crucial to recognize and understand unhealthy ones that may exacerbate anger issues.

1. Suppression of Emotions: Suppressing emotions, or bottling them up, is a common but unhealthy coping mechanism. This approach may provide temporary relief, but it often leads to an eventual eruption of intense emotions.

2. Escapism: Engaging in activities solely to escape reality, such as excessive screen time or substance use, can become a maladaptive coping mechanism. While it may offer a temporary reprieve, it does not address the underlying issues.

3. Blame and Projection: Projecting one's emotions onto others or external circumstances is another unhealthy coping mechanism. This deflective strategy prevents self-reflection and inhibits personal growth.

The Transformative Power of Healthy Coping Mechanisms

Developing healthy coping mechanisms is not only about managing anger but also about fostering emotional intelligence and long-term well-being. These strategies empower parents to respond to challenges with resilience, intentionality, and a deeper understanding of their emotions.

1. Emotional Regulation Techniques: Healthy coping mechanisms include emotional regulation techniques, such as deep breathing, mindfulness, and grounding exercises. These practices enable parents to manage the intensity of emotions and respond thoughtfully.

2. Effective Communication: Cultivating healthy communication skills is a transformative coping mechanism. Expressing emotions assertively, actively

listening, and using "I" statements create an environment of openness and understanding.

Strategies for Developing Healthy Coping Mechanisms

The journey toward healthy coping mechanisms involves intentional effort and a commitment to personal growth. Here are strategies that empower parents to cultivate constructive ways of managing anger and stress.

1. Self-Reflection: Engaging in regular self-reflection is a cornerstone of developing healthy coping mechanisms. This introspective practice allows parents to identify patterns, triggers, and the effectiveness of their current coping strategies.

2. Seeking Professional Guidance: Therapists, counselors, or support groups provide valuable insights and guidance in developing healthy coping mechanisms. Professional intervention offers tailored

strategies and a safe space for exploring and refining coping mechanisms.

3. Mindfulness Practices: Mindfulness, as explored in previous chapters, is a multifaceted coping mechanism. Integrating mindfulness practices into daily life enhances self-awareness, emotional regulation, and the capacity for intentional responses.

Coping Mechanisms Tailored for Parenting

Parenting introduces a unique set of stressors and challenges, necessitating coping mechanisms that are tailored to the demands of this role.

1. Time Management Strategies: Developing effective time management skills is a practical coping mechanism for parents. Prioritizing tasks, setting realistic goals, and embracing flexibility alleviate the stress associated with balancing parental responsibilities.

2. Parental Support Networks: Building a supportive network of fellow parents provides a valuable emotional outlet. Sharing experiences, seeking advice, and receiving empathy contribute to a sense of camaraderie and diminish the isolation often felt in parenting.

Emotional Expression and Catharsis

Healthy coping mechanisms embrace the expression of emotions rather than their suppression. Emotional catharsis, or the release of pent-up feelings, is a pivotal aspect of constructive coping.

1. Journaling and Artistic Expression: Journaling serves as a therapeutic outlet for emotional expression. Writing down thoughts and emotions provides a structured means of processing challenges. Similarly, engaging in artistic expression, whether through drawing, painting, or other creative outlets, can be a cathartic release.

2. Physical Activity and Exercise: Incorporating regular physical activity into the routine is a powerful coping mechanism. Exercise not only promotes physical health but also releases endorphins, the body's natural mood lifters, contributing to emotional well-being.

Transformative Effects on Parent-Child Relationships

The adoption of healthy coping mechanisms extends beyond individual well-being to influence the parent-child dynamic. Parents who model constructive coping strategies contribute to a positive emotional climate within the family.

1. Teaching Emotional Regulation: Parents serve as emotional guides for their children. Modeling healthy coping mechanisms teaches children the importance of emotional regulation and equips them with

valuable skills for navigating their own emotions.

2. Creating a Supportive Environment: A household where healthy coping mechanisms are practiced fosters a supportive environment. Children, observing their parents' resilience and intentionality, learn to approach challenges with adaptability and emotional intelligence.

Long-Term Benefits of Healthy Coping Mechanisms

The impact of cultivating healthy coping mechanisms extends far beyond immediate stress relief. It lays the foundation for sustained emotional well-being and personal growth.

1. Building Emotional Resilience: Healthy coping mechanisms contribute to the development of emotional resilience. Parents who navigate challenges with constructive strategies build a robust

emotional foundation that withstands the complexities of parenthood.

2. Enhancing Problem-Solving Skills: Effective coping mechanisms are intertwined with problem-solving skills. Parents who approach challenges with a solution-oriented mindset not only manage anger more effectively but also impart valuable problem-solving skills to their children.

In the mosaic of parenthood, the cultivation of healthy coping mechanisms emerges as a transformative journey—one that empowers parents to be the architects of their emotional responses, fostering resilience and creating a harmonious family dynamic. By identifying and replacing unhealthy coping mechanisms, parents embark on a path of self-discovery, personal growth, and the legacy of emotional well-being that reverberates through the generations.

5.1.1 Deep Breathing Exercises

In the tumultuous journey of parenthood, where emotions ebb and flow like a tempest, the art of deep breathing emerges as a potent elixir—an invaluable tool in the pursuit of anger management mastery. This chapter delves into the transformative power of deep breathing exercises, exploring how they empower parents to be the masters of their emotions, fostering resilience, and cultivating a serene family environment.

The Physiology of Deep Breathing

Deep breathing, also known as diaphragmatic or abdominal breathing, engages the diaphragm—a dome-shaped muscle separating the chest and abdomen. Unlike shallow chest breathing, which is often associated with stress, deep breathing activates the diaphragm, promoting a cascade of physiological benefits.

1. Activating the Relaxation Response: Deep breathing triggers the body's relaxation

response, activating the parasympathetic nervous system. This counteracts the fight-or-flight response, inducing a state of calmness and reducing the physiological markers of stress.

2. Oxygenating the Body: Deep breaths increase the intake of oxygen, enriching the bloodstream and promoting optimal functioning of vital organs. Enhanced oxygenation contributes to increased energy levels and mental clarity.

Deep Breathing as an Anchor in Anger Management

In the realm of anger management, deep breathing serves as a steadfast anchor—a grounding practice that interrupts the cycle of escalating emotions and provides parents with a sanctuary of calm amidst the storm.

1. Interrupting the Automatic Response:
Anger often triggers automatic, impulsive reactions. Deep breathing introduces a

deliberate pause, disrupting the automatic response and creating space for a more intentional and measured reaction.

2. Calming the Emotional Storm: Deep breathing acts as a balm for emotional turbulence. By calming the physiological response to anger, it sets the stage for a clearer mindset, enabling parents to navigate challenges with composure.

Practical Deep Breathing Techniques

The beauty of deep breathing lies in its accessibility and simplicity. Integrating these techniques into daily life empowers parents to foster emotional regulation and resilience.

1. Diaphragmatic Breathing: Begin by finding a comfortable, quiet space. Inhale deeply through the nose, allowing the diaphragm to expand fully. Exhale slowly through pursed lips, engaging the abdominal muscles. Repeat this cycle for several breaths, gradually extending the duration.

2. 4-7-8 Breathing Technique: Popularized by Dr. Andrew Weil, the 4-7-8 technique involves inhaling quietly through the nose for a count of four, holding the breath for a count of seven, and exhaling audibly through the mouth for a count of eight. This rhythmic pattern promotes relaxation and balance.

Integrating Deep Breathing into Daily Life

The transformative impact of deep breathing extends beyond designated practice sessions. Integrating this technique into daily life establishes it as a natural and accessible resource for emotional well-being.

1. Morning Rituals: Begin the day with a few minutes of deep breathing. This sets a positive tone, fostering a sense of calm and mindfulness that can influence the entire day.

2. Transition Moments: Use transition moments, such as before entering or exiting the home, to practice deep breathing. This intentional pause creates a buffer between different environments, allowing parents to approach each situation with greater equilibrium.

Deep Breathing for Real-Time Anger Management

The efficacy of deep breathing shines in real-time anger management scenarios. When faced with a triggering situation, these exercises become immediate allies, guiding parents towards measured responses.

1. The "Take Five" Approach: When anger surfaces, take five intentional deep breaths before responding. This brief pause provides the necessary distance from the initial emotional surge, enabling a more thoughtful and controlled reaction.

2. Mindful Breathing During Conflict: In the midst of a conflict, practice mindful breathing to anchor yourself in the present moment. Focus on the sensation of each breath, allowing it to serve as a reminder to respond with intentionality rather than react impulsively.

Incorporating Visualization with Deep Breathing

Combining deep breathing with visualization enhances its impact, creating a holistic approach to anger management.

1. Imagery of Release: As you exhale deeply, visualize releasing pent-up tension and frustration. Picture the negative emotions dissipating with each breath, leaving space for a renewed sense of calm.

2. Cleansing Breath: Envision the inhalation as a cleansing process, drawing in positive energy and clarity. As you exhale, visualize

expelling stress and negativity, leaving a purified emotional state.

Progressive Deep Breathing Practices

As parents become adept at basic deep breathing, progressive practices can be introduced to deepen the benefits.

1. Extended Breath Holds: Gradually extend the duration of breath holds in the 4-7-8 technique. This challenges the body's capacity for relaxation, promoting resilience in the face of stressors.

2. Layered Breathing Exercises: Combine deep breathing with other relaxation techniques, such as progressive muscle relaxation or guided imagery. This layered approach enhances the overall impact, fostering a comprehensive sense of well-being.

The Role of Consistency in Deep Breathing Practices

The transformative power of deep breathing unfolds over time, emphasizing the importance of consistency.

1. Establishing a Routine: Incorporate deep breathing into daily routines, creating a consistent practice. Whether during moments of solitude, while commuting, or before bedtime, regularity enhances the effectiveness of deep breathing as a coping mechanism.

2. Family Practice Sessions: Introduce deep breathing as a family practice. Gather together for brief sessions, fostering a shared commitment to emotional well-being. This not only benefits individual family members

but also contributes to a harmonious household atmosphere.

Professional Guidance and Support

For parents facing persistent challenges in anger management or those seeking to deepen their practice, seeking professional guidance can provide invaluable support.

1. Therapeutic Interventions: Therapists specializing in anger management can incorporate deep breathing into therapeutic interventions. These professionals guide parents through the exploration of triggers and the development of personalized coping strategies.

2. Support Groups: Participating in support groups offers a communal space for sharing experiences and learning from others. These groups often include discussions on coping

mechanisms, providing additional insights and encouragement.

The Long-Term Legacy of Deep Breathing

In the narrative of parenthood, deep breathing stands as a timeless legacy—an enduring gift that reverberates through the generations. By mastering the art of intentional breath, parents cultivate emotional resilience, nurture a serene family environment, and embark on a journey of self-discovery that shapes not only their own well-being but also the emotional landscape of the family for years to come.

5.1.2 Visualization Techniques

In the intricate canvas of parenthood, where emotions paint vibrant strokes across the daily landscape, the art of visualization emerges as a potent brush—an exquisite tool in the pursuit of anger management mastery. This chapter explores the transformative power of visualization techniques, offering parents a palette to craft a serene emotional landscape and become true masters of their emotions.

The Essence of Visualization

Visualization, also known as mental imagery or guided imagery, is a powerful technique that involves creating vivid mental images. In the realm of anger management, visualization becomes a dynamic practice, enabling parents to sculpt the contours of their emotional responses and foster a tranquil family environment.

1. Harnessing the Power of Imagination: Visualization taps into the vast reservoir of imagination. By conjuring mental images that evoke calmness and positivity, parents engage their imaginative faculties to influence their emotional state positively.

2. Creating a Mental Sanctuary: Visualization empowers parents to create mental sanctuaries—a haven of tranquility within their minds. These imagined spaces become retreats where they can navigate the storms of anger with grace and composure.

The Interplay Between Mind and Emotion

Visualization operates at the intersection of the mind and emotions, offering a bridge between thought and feeling.

1. Shaping Emotional Responses: Through visualization, parents can rehearse positive emotional responses to potential triggers. This mental rehearsal contributes to the rewiring of automatic reactions, fostering intentional and measured responses.

2. Impact on Stress Reduction: Visualization serves as a stress reduction tool. As parents immerse themselves in calming images, the mind sends signals to the body to relax,

activating the parasympathetic nervous system and mitigating the physiological markers of stress.

Practical Visualization Techniques

Visualization techniques are versatile and adaptable, allowing parents to tailor the practice to their unique preferences and circumstances.

1. Guided Imagery Scripts: Utilize guided imagery scripts that lead parents through a series of calming scenes. These scripts often include vivid descriptions of serene landscapes, soothing sounds, and scenarios that evoke relaxation.

2. Personalized Mental Imagery: Craft personalized mental images that hold specific calming associations. This could range from imagining a tranquil beach at sunset to envisioning a peaceful meadow. The key is to create mental images that

resonate with individual preferences and bring about a sense of calm.

Integrating Visualization into Daily Life

The efficacy of visualization lies in its integration into the fabric of daily life, becoming a seamless thread woven into routine activities.

1. Morning Visualization Rituals: Begin the day with a brief visualization session. Picture the day unfolding smoothly, envisioning positive interactions with children, and navigating challenges with calmness. This sets a positive tone for the day ahead.

2. Visualization Before Challenging Situations: Prior to potentially challenging situations, take a moment for visualization. Picture yourself responding to the situation with patience and understanding. This pre-emptive practice prepares the mind for intentional responses.

Real-Time Visualization for Anger Management

The real-time application of visualization becomes a dynamic tool in the face of anger triggers, guiding parents toward a composed and intentional response.

1. The "Pause and Picture" Technique: When anger begins to surface, initiate a brief pause. Close your eyes and picture a calming image—a place, a scene, or an experience that brings about a sense of tranquility. This mental break interrupts the automatic escalation of emotions.

2. Visualizing Positive Outcomes: Envision positive outcomes in challenging situations. Picture conflicts resolving amicably, and visualize the restoration of harmony within the family. This optimistic mental imagery shapes the emotional landscape during moments of potential conflict.

Progressive Visualization Practices

As parents become adept at basic visualization techniques, progressive practices can deepen the impact and foster sustained emotional well-being.

1. Scenario Rehearsal: Engage in scenario rehearsal through visualization. Picture specific situations that typically trigger anger and visualize yourself responding with patience and empathy. This mental rehearsal enhances preparedness for real-life scenarios.

2. Emotion-Focused Visualization: Direct visualization towards specific emotions. Picture a scenario that typically elicits anger and visualize transforming that emotion into patience, understanding, or another positive response. This focused practice enhances emotional intelligence.

Guided Group Visualization Sessions

To enhance the impact of visualization, consider incorporating guided group sessions, fostering shared moments of calmness within the family.

1. Family Visualization Sessions: Gather as a family for brief visualization sessions. This collective practice not only enhances individual emotional well-being but also contributes to a shared sense of tranquility within the household.

2. Guided Group Imagery: Engage in guided imagery as a family. Choose scenarios that resonate with everyone, fostering a sense of unity and shared positive experiences. This collective visualization contributes to the creation of a harmonious family dynamic.

Professional Guidance and Visualization

For parents seeking to deepen their practice or those facing persistent challenges, professional guidance can provide valuable support.

1. Therapeutic Visualization Techniques:
Therapists specializing in anger
management often incorporate visualization
techniques into therapeutic interventions.
These professionals guide parents through
tailored visualization practices, addressing
individual triggers and responses.

2. Visualization-Based Workshops:
Participate in visualization-based workshops
or support groups. These settings provide a
structured environment for learning and
practicing visualization techniques, often
including guided sessions and opportunities
for shared experiences.

The Timeless Legacy of Visualization

In the tapestry of parenthood, visualization
stands as a timeless legacy—a brushstroke
of tranquility that echoes through the
generations. By harnessing the power of
mental imagery, parents cultivate emotional
resilience, nurture a serene family

environment, and embark on a journey of self-discovery that shapes not only their own well-being but also the emotional landscape of the family for years to come. Through the canvas of visualization, parents paint a legacy of calmness, intentionality, and emotional mastery—a masterpiece that endures through the ebbs and flows of family life.

5.2 Effective Communication Skills

In the intricate dance of parenthood, where emotions intertwine and clashes are inevitable, the mastery of effective communication becomes a beacon—an invaluable tool in the pursuit of anger management. This chapter explores the transformative power of communication skills, offering parents a roadmap to navigate the complexities of emotions, foster understanding, and create a harmonious family dynamic.

The Crucial Role of Effective Communication

Effective communication is the linchpin of healthy relationships, and within the realm of parenting, its significance amplifies. It becomes a nuanced dance of expressing emotions, actively listening, and choosing words with intentionality.

1. Definition of Effective Communication: Effective communication goes beyond the exchange of words. It involves the art of conveying thoughts, emotions, and needs in a way that is clear, respectful, and conducive to understanding.

2. Impact on Parental Well-Being: The quality of communication directly influences parental well-being. Effective communication acts as a bridge, fostering connection, and mitigating potential conflicts that may lead to anger.

The Dynamics of Anger and Communication

Understanding the interplay between anger and communication is essential for parents seeking mastery over their emotional responses.

1. The Escalation of Anger through Poor Communication: Ineffective communication often acts as fuel for the fire of anger. Misunderstandings, unexpressed emotions, and a lack of clarity can escalate tension and give rise to unnecessary conflicts.

2. Communication as a Tool for Anger Management: Conversely, effective communication serves as a powerful tool in the arsenal of anger management. It enables parents to express their emotions constructively, fosters empathy, and cultivates an environment where conflicts can be resolved amicably.

Core Elements of Effective Communication

Effective communication is a multifaceted skill that encompasses several core elements.

1. Active Listening: The foundation of effective communication lies in active listening. This involves fully focusing on the speaker, withholding judgment, and providing feedback to ensure understanding.

2. Expressing Emotions Assertively: Communicating emotions assertively involves expressing feelings in a direct yet respectful manner. This allows parents to convey their emotional state without resorting to aggression or blame.

Strategies for Developing Effective Communication Skills

The journey toward effective communication is an ongoing process that requires intentional effort and self-reflection.

1.   Reflective   Self-Expression: Before engaging in a conversation, take a moment for reflective self-expression. Identify the emotions at play and consider the desired outcome of the communication. This self-awareness lays the groundwork for intentional expression.

2. Mindful Speech: Integrate mindfulness into speech by choosing words with care. Mindful speech involves considering the impact of words on the listener and expressing thoughts with clarity and compassion.

Conflict Resolution through Effective Communication

Conflict is an inevitable part of family life, but effective communication serves as a compass, guiding parents toward resolution rather than escalation.

1. The "I" Statements Technique: Utilize "I" statements to express feelings and needs

without assigning blame. For example, instead of saying, "You always make me angry," one might say, "I feel frustrated when..."

2. Seeking Understanding Through Questions: When faced with conflicting perspectives, seek understanding through open-ended questions. This not only demonstrates a willingness to listen but also fosters an environment where differing opinions can be explored constructively.

Practical Application of Communication Skills in Anger Management

The real-time application of communication skills is pivotal during moments of heightened emotions.

1. The Pause-and-Reflect Approach: When anger surfaces, initiate a pause before responding. Reflect on the emotions at play and consider how they can be expressed in a

way that fosters understanding rather than escalation.

2. De-escalation Through Verbal Cues: Develop verbal cues that signal a commitment to de-escalation. Phrases like "Let's take a moment to understand each other" or "I want to hear your perspective" pave the way for constructive communication.

Nonverbal Communication in Anger Management

Nonverbal cues are as influential as words in the realm of communication. Being attuned to and intentional about nonverbal communication enhances the effectiveness of the overall message.

1. Body Language and Facial Expressions: Pay attention to body language and facial expressions. An open and relaxed posture communicates receptiveness, while tension

and aggressive gestures may escalate conflict.

2. Tone of Voice: The tone of voice can convey more than the words themselves. Strive for a calm and even tone, avoiding harshness or raised volume, which can trigger defensive reactions.

Seeking Professional Guidance for Communication Enhancement

For parents navigating persistent challenges in communication, seeking professional guidance can provide valuable insights and support.

1. Family Therapy Sessions: Family therapy sessions offer a structured environment for improving communication dynamics. Therapists can identify patterns, provide strategies for more effective communication,

and guide the family toward conflict resolution.

2. Communication Workshops: Participate in communication workshops or support groups. These settings often provide practical tools, role-playing exercises, and shared experiences that contribute to enhanced communication skills.

The Long-Term Impact of Effective Communication

The mastery of effective communication is a gift that reverberates through the generations—a legacy of understanding, empathy, and harmonious relationships.

1. Building Emotional Resilience in Children: Parents who model effective communication skills impart valuable lessons to their children. This legacy equips the younger generation with the tools to

navigate emotions, resolve conflicts, and build emotional resilience.

2. Fostering a Positive Family Dynamic: A family built on effective communication becomes a sanctuary of understanding and support. As family members learn to express themselves authentically and listen empathetically, the foundation for a positive and harmonious dynamic is laid.

In the intricate tapestry of parenthood, effective communication emerges as a guiding thread—a transformative skill that empowers parents to navigate the complexities of emotions, resolve conflicts, and create a harmonious family environment. By mastering the art of harmonious dialogue, parents not only enhance their own well-being but also weave a legacy of understanding and connection that resonates through the generations, fostering resilient and emotionally intelligent individuals within the family fold.

5.2.1 Active Listening

In the symphony of parenthood, where emotions crescendo and decrescendo, the art of active listening emerges as a silent yet powerful conductor—an essential skill in the pursuit of anger management mastery. This chapter explores the transformative power of active listening, unveiling how it empowers parents to navigate the complexities of emotions, build connection, and orchestrate a harmonious family dynamic.

The Essence of Active Listening

Active listening is more than the act of hearing words; it is a dynamic and engaged process of truly understanding the speaker. In the context of anger management, active listening becomes a bridge, fostering empathy and creating a space for authentic communication.

1. Definition of Active Listening: Active listening involves fully concentrating, understanding, responding, and remembering what is being said. It goes beyond passively hearing words, delving into the emotional undercurrents and unspoken nuances.

2. Impact on Parental Well-Being: The quality of communication is intricately tied to parental well-being. Active listening acts as a conduit for understanding, diminishing misunderstandings, and providing a platform for expressing emotions constructively.

Active Listening Dynamics in Anger Management

Understanding how active listening intersects with anger management is crucial for parents seeking mastery over their emotional responses.

1. Defusing Tension Through Presence: The mere act of being present and fully attentive

can defuse tension. Active listening signals a willingness to understand, creating an environment where anger can be expressed without fear of judgment.

2. Empathy as a Buffer for Anger: Active listening is a channel for empathy. When parents actively listen, they step into the emotional shoes of the speaker, building a bridge of understanding that serves as a buffer against escalating anger.

Core Elements of Active Listening

Active listening involves a set of key elements that transform it from a passive activity into a dynamic and intentional skill.

1. Reflective Responses: Responding reflectively involves paraphrasing or summarizing the speaker's words. This not only confirms understanding but also allows the speaker to clarify or expand on their thoughts.

2. Nonverbal Cues: Nonverbal cues, such as maintaining eye contact, nodding, and adopting an open and engaged posture, signal active involvement in the conversation. These cues convey receptiveness and support.

Strategies for Developing Active Listening Skills

The journey toward active listening mastery requires intentional effort and a commitment to ongoing improvement.

1. Mindful Presence: Practice mindful presence during conversations. Set aside distractions, turn off electronic devices, and focus entirely on the speaker. Mindful presence creates a conducive space for active listening.

2. Suppressing the Urge to Interrupt: It is common to feel the urge to interrupt with one's thoughts or responses. Suppressing this urge and allowing the speaker to express themselves fully is a fundamental aspect of active listening.

Active Listening as a Conflict Resolution Tool

In the realm of anger management, active listening serves as a potent tool for de-escalating conflicts and fostering resolution.

1. The Power of Validation: Validating the speaker's feelings is a cornerstone of active listening. Acknowledging emotions without judgment or defensiveness validates the speaker's experience, reducing the intensity of anger.

2. Uncovering Root Issues Through Probing Questions: Probing questions that seek to understand the root issues behind expressed emotions contribute to conflict resolution. Active listening involves delving into the underlying causes of anger and addressing them collaboratively.

Real-Time Application of Active Listening in Anger Management

The real-time application of active listening becomes pivotal during moments of heightened emotions.

1. The "Pause and Listen" Approach: When anger begins to surface, initiate a pause. Encourage the speaker to share their thoughts and feelings. This deliberate pause interrupts the automatic escalation of emotions, creating space for understanding.

2. Expressing Empathy Through Verbal Cues: Verbal cues that express empathy,

such as "I understand," or "Tell me more about how you're feeling," convey a genuine desire to comprehend the speaker's perspective. This empathetic engagement de-escalates anger and fosters connection.

Nonverbal Components of Active Listening

Beyond words, nonverbal components contribute significantly to the effectiveness of active listening.

1. Mirroring Emotions: Nonverbal mirroring involves reflecting the speaker's emotions through facial expressions and body language. This nonverbal alignment reinforces the understanding of the speaker's emotional state.

2. Maintaining Calm Body Language: Active listening is accentuated by

maintaining calm and open body language. Avoiding defensive postures or expressions communicates receptivity and creates an environment conducive to open communication.

Seeking Professional Guidance for Active Listening Enhancement

For parents seeking to deepen their active listening skills or facing persistent challenges, seeking professional guidance can offer valuable insights.

1. Family Counseling Sessions: Family counseling sessions provide a structured environment for improving communication dynamics. Therapists can observe and guide active listening practices, fostering a more empathetic and understanding family dynamic.

2. Communication Skills Workshops: Participate in communication skills workshops or support groups. These settings often include role-playing exercises, practical tools, and shared experiences that contribute to enhanced active listening skills.

The Long-Term Legacy of Active Listening

The mastery of active listening is a gift that resonates through the generations—a legacy of understanding, empathy, and harmonious relationships.

1. Building Emotional Intelligence in Children: Parents who model active listening skills contribute significantly to the emotional intelligence of their children. This legacy equips the younger generation with the ability to navigate emotions, communicate effectively, and build meaningful connections.

2. Fostering a Culture of Open Communication: A family rooted in active listening becomes a haven of open communication. As family members learn to listen and be heard, the foundation for a positive and harmonious dynamic is laid, shaping the family culture for years to come. In the symphony of parenthood, active listening emerges as a silent conductor—an invisible force that harmonizes emotions, defuses conflicts, and creates a family dynamic rooted in understanding and connection. By mastering the art of active listening, parents not only enhance their own well-being but also weave a legacy of empathy and emotional mastery that reverberates through the family tapestry. In the quietude of active listening, parents find the power to transform anger into understanding and discord into harmony—a silent symphony that resonates through the generations.

5.2.2 Expressing Emotions Constructively

In the intricate dance of parenthood, where emotions sway like the changing tides, the art of expressing emotions constructively emerges as a transformative brushstroke—an essential skill in the pursuit of anger management mastery. This chapter delves into the significance of constructive emotional expression, exploring how it empowers parents to navigate the complexities of anger, foster connection, and cultivate a harmonious family environment.

The Role of Emotional Expression in Anger Management

Emotions are an inherent aspect of the human experience, and parents, in the course of raising children, often find themselves contending with a spectrum of emotions, including anger. Constructive emotional expression becomes the linchpin in converting the potent energy of anger into a force for positive change.

1.   Defining   Constructive   Emotional Expression: Constructive   emotional expression involves communicating one's feelings in a way that is respectful, clear, and conducive to understanding. It provides a healthy outlet for the release of pent-up emotions, preventing the escalation of anger.

2. Impact on Parental Well-Being: The ability to express emotions constructively directly influences parental well-being. It serves as a release valve, preventing the buildup of emotional pressure that may lead to explosive anger, and fosters an environment where emotions are acknowledged and addressed.

Dynamics of Anger and Emotional Expression

Understanding how anger and emotional expression intersect is essential for parents seeking mastery over their emotional responses.

1. Unpacking Anger Triggers: Constructive emotional expression involves unpacking the triggers of anger. It requires introspection to identify the root causes, enabling parents to address underlying issues rather than reacting to surface-level provocations.

2. Embracing Vulnerability: Constructive emotional expression requires embracing vulnerability. It involves being open about one's feelings without succumbing to the need for defensiveness or blame. This vulnerability creates a space for authentic communication.

Core Elements of Constructive Emotional Expression

Constructive emotional expression is a nuanced skill that encompasses several key elements.

1. Clear Communication of Feelings: The foundation of constructive emotional

expression lies in the clear communication of feelings. Articulating emotions with precision fosters understanding and prevents misinterpretation.

2. Assertive, Not Aggressive, Expression: Constructive emotional expression is assertive, not aggressive. It involves expressing feelings firmly and directly without resorting to blaming language or confrontational behavior.

Strategies for Developing Constructive Emotional Expression

The journey toward mastering constructive emotional expression requires intentional effort and a commitment to ongoing self-improvement.

1. Journaling as a Reflective Tool: Journaling provides a private space for reflecting on emotions. Writing down feelings allows parents to process and

organize their thoughts before engaging in constructive conversations.

2. Mindful Self-Reflection: Incorporate mindful self-reflection into daily routines. Before responding to a potentially triggering situation, take a moment to assess and understand your emotions. This mindfulness enhances the clarity of emotional expression.

Constructive Emotional Expression as a Conflict Resolution Tool

In the realm of anger management, constructive emotional expression serves as a powerful tool for resolving conflicts and fostering understanding.

1. Using "I" Statements: Constructive emotional expression often involves using "I" statements to communicate feelings. For example, saying, "I feel frustrated when..." avoids placing blame on others and focuses on personal emotions and experiences.

2. Expressing Needs and Desires: Constructive emotional expression extends to expressing needs and desires. Clearly communicating what is needed or desired allows for collaborative problem-solving and prevents the accumulation of unmet expectations.

Real-Time Application of Constructive Emotional Expression in Anger Management

The real-time application of constructive emotional expression becomes pivotal during moments of heightened emotions.

1. The Pause-and-Express Approach: When anger surfaces, initiate a brief pause. Use this time to reflect on the emotions at play and express them constructively. This deliberate pause interrupts the automatic escalation of emotions and creates space for understanding.

2. Framing Emotions with Positive Intent: Constructive emotional expression involves framing emotions with positive intent. Instead of framing a grievance as an accusation, express it as a desire for improvement or understanding. This approach encourages collaboration rather than defensiveness.

Nonverbal Components of Constructive Emotional Expression

Beyond words, nonverbal components contribute significantly to the effectiveness of constructive emotional expression.

1. Facial Expressions and Body Language: Nonverbal cues, such as facial expressions and body language, play a crucial role. A calm and open demeanor conveys receptivity, while aggressive or defensive postures may hinder constructive communication.

2. Tone of Voice: The tone of voice can influence the reception of emotional expression. Maintaining a calm and even tone prevents the communication of anger from escalating into a confrontational exchange.

Seeking Professional Guidance for Constructive Emotional Expression

For parents seeking to deepen their skills in constructive emotional expression or facing persistent challenges, seeking professional guidance can offer valuable insights.

1. Individual or Family Counseling: Individual or family counseling sessions provide a structured environment for improving emotional expression dynamics. Therapists can observe and guide constructive emotional expression practices, fostering a more empathetic and understanding family dynamic.

2. Emotional Intelligence Workshops: Participate in emotional intelligence workshops or support groups. These settings often include role-playing exercises, practical tools, and shared experiences that contribute to enhanced constructive emotional expression skills.

The Long-Term Impact of Constructive Emotional Expression

The mastery of constructive emotional expression is a gift that resonates through the generations—a legacy of emotional intelligence, understanding, and harmonious relationships.

1. Building Emotional Resilience in Children: Parents who model constructive emotional expression contribute significantly to the emotional resilience of their children. This legacy equips the younger generation with the tools to navigate emotions, express themselves

effectively, and build meaningful connections.

2. Fostering a Culture of Emotional Openness: A family rooted in constructive emotional expression becomes a sanctuary of emotional openness. As family members learn to express and respond to emotions constructively, the foundation for a positive and harmonious dynamic is laid, shaping the family culture for years to come.

In the rich tapestry of parenthood, constructive emotional expression emerges as an expressive brushstroke—a vibrant hue that transforms the canvas of emotions. By mastering the art of expressing emotions constructively, parents not only enhance their own well-being but also weave a legacy of emotional intelligence and connection that resonates through the family tapestry. In the dance of constructive emotional expression, parents find the power to transform anger into understanding, conflicts into opportunities for growth, and the family dynamic into a symphony of harmonious relationships—a masterpiece that endures through the ebbs and flows of family life.

Chapter 6: Building Stronger Parent-Child Relationships

6.1 Repairing and Rebuilding Trust

In the complex terrain of parenthood, where emotions run deep and clashes are inevitable, the art of repairing and rebuilding trust emerges as a profound journey—a crucial aspect in the pursuit of anger management mastery. This chapter delves into the significance of trust repair, exploring how parents can navigate the aftermath of anger, rebuild fractured connections, and cultivate a resilient and harmonious family environment.

The Fragility of Trust in Parenting

Trust is the bedrock of any relationship, and within the parent-child dynamic, it takes on heightened significance. When anger erupts and emotions escalate, trust can suffer collateral damage. Acknowledging the fragility of trust becomes the first step in its repair.

1. Defining Trust Repair: Trust repair involves intentional actions aimed at rebuilding the foundation of trust that may have been compromised. It requires humility, accountability, and a commitment to change.

2. Impact on Parental Well-Being: The state of trust in the parent-child relationship directly influences parental well-being. Trust repair is not only vital for the child's emotional security but also for the parent's sense of efficacy and fulfillment in their role.

Dynamics of Trust and Anger

Understanding the intricate dynamics between trust and anger is essential for parents seeking mastery over their emotional responses.

1. Trust Erosion through Anger: Uncontrolled anger can erode trust. When children witness parents expressing anger in ways that are hurtful or frightening, it shakes the foundation of the trust they place in their caregivers.

2. Rebuilding Trust as a Healing Process: Rebuilding trust is a healing process. It involves acknowledging the impact of anger on the parent-child relationship and taking deliberate steps to mend the ruptured bonds.

Core Elements of Trust Repair

Trust repair is a nuanced process that involves specific elements aimed at rebuilding the fractured bridge of trust.

1. Accountability for Actions: The foundation of trust repair lies in accountability. Parents must take ownership of their actions and acknowledge the impact of their anger on the child. This honesty forms the cornerstone of trust rebuilding.

2. Consistent Positive Change: Trust is rebuilt through consistent positive change. Parents must demonstrate, through their actions, a commitment to managing anger more effectively and creating a nurturing and secure environment for their child.

Strategies for Trust Repair in Anger Management

The journey toward rebuilding trust is multifaceted, requiring intentional efforts and ongoing commitment.

1. Open Communication: Trust repair involves open communication. Parents should create a safe space for their children to express their feelings and concerns. Open dialogue fosters understanding and paves the way for rebuilding trust.

2. Establishing Clear Boundaries: Trust rebuilding requires the establishment of clear boundaries. Parents should define acceptable and unacceptable behavior,

creating a framework that supports emotional safety within the family.

Trust Repair as a Continuous Process

Trust repair is not a one-time fix but a continuous process that requires sustained effort and commitment.

1. Patience and Understanding: Parents must exercise patience and understanding. Rebuilding trust is a gradual process, and children may need time to heal from the impact of anger. Patiently supporting them through this journey is essential.

2. Regular Check-Ins: Regular check-ins create opportunities for ongoing communication. Parents should consistently check in with their children, expressing a genuine interest in their feelings and experiences. These regular interactions contribute to the rebuilding of trust.

Real-Time Application of Trust Repair in Anger Management

The real-time application of trust repair becomes pivotal during moments of potential conflict or anger.

1. Immediate Acknowledgment and Apology: When anger results in a breach of trust, immediate acknowledgment and apology are crucial. Parents should promptly recognize the impact of their actions, apologize sincerely, and express a commitment to positive change.

2. Consistent Positive Reinforcement: Trust repair involves consistent positive reinforcement. Parents should actively seek opportunities to reinforce positive behaviors, fostering an environment where trust can gradually be rebuilt.

Nonverbal Components of Trust Repair

Beyond words, nonverbal components contribute significantly to the effectiveness of trust repair.

1. Demonstrating Empathy: Nonverbal cues, such as facial expressions and body language, play a significant role in demonstrating empathy. Parents should convey genuine remorse and understanding through their nonverbal communication.

2. Affection and Reassurance: Physical affection and reassurance are powerful nonverbal tools in trust repair. Hugs, comforting gestures, and verbal reassurances contribute to a sense of safety and reaffirmation of the parent-child bond.

Seeking Professional Guidance for Trust Repair

For parents navigating persistent challenges in trust repair, seeking professional guidance can provide valuable support.

1. Family Counseling: Family counseling sessions offer a structured environment for addressing trust issues. Therapists can guide parents and children through the process of rebuilding trust, facilitating open communication and understanding.

2. Parenting Support Groups: Participating in parenting support groups provides a communal space for sharing experiences and learning from others. These groups often offer insights and strategies for effective trust repair within the parent-child relationship.

The Long-Term Impact of Trust Repair

The mastery of trust repair is a gift that echoes through the generations—a legacy of resilience, understanding, and harmonious relationships.

1. Building Emotional Resilience in Children: Parents who navigate the journey of trust repair with authenticity and commitment contribute significantly to the emotional resilience of their children. This legacy equips the younger generation with the tools to navigate challenges, express emotions, and build healthy relationships.

2. Fostering a Culture of Forgiveness: A family rooted in trust repair becomes a testament to the power of forgiveness. As parents model accountability, positive change, and the capacity for healing, they cultivate a culture of forgiveness that transcends conflicts and strengthens the family bond.

In the intricate tapestry of parenthood, trust repair emerges as a transformative thread—a testament to the resilience of familial bonds. By mastering the art of rebuilding trust after anger, parents not only enhance their own well-being but also weave a legacy of resilience, understanding, and connection that reverberates through the family tapestry. In the deliberate steps of trust repair, parents find the power to transform conflict into growth, anger into constructive change, and fractured connections into resilient bonds that endure through the trials of family life.

6.1.1 Apologizing and Making Amends

In the intricate dance of parenthood, where emotions ebb and flow, the art of apologizing and making amends emerges as a profound and transformative practice—an indispensable skill in the pursuit of anger management mastery. This chapter explores the significance of offering genuine apologies and making meaningful amends, revealing how parents can navigate the aftermath of anger, foster healing, and cultivate a resilient and harmonious family environment.

The Power of Apology in Parenting

Apologizing is a fundamental aspect of healthy communication, and within the parent-child dynamic, it takes on heightened significance. When anger surfaces and emotions run high, the ability to offer a sincere apology becomes a bridge to healing.

1. Defining a Genuine Apology: A genuine apology involves expressing remorse for one's actions, acknowledging the impact on others, and demonstrating a commitment to positive change. It goes beyond mere words, encompassing a heartfelt recognition of the pain caused.

2. Impact on Parental Well-Being: The act of apologizing directly influences parental well-being. It not only fosters emotional

release and relief for the parent but also sets the stage for rebuilding trust and connection within the family.

Dynamics of Apology and Anger

Understanding how apology dynamics intersect with anger is crucial for parents seeking mastery over their emotional responses.

1. Apology as a Reset Button: Offering a sincere apology serves as a reset button. It interrupts the cycle of anger, signaling a willingness to acknowledge mistakes and fostering an environment conducive to healing.

2. Healing Wounds Through Apology: Apology is a healing balm for emotional wounds. It provides an opportunity for both parent and child to process and release negative emotions, paving the way for a renewed sense of understanding.

Core Elements of a Genuine Apology

A genuine apology is a nuanced practice that involves specific elements aimed at fostering healing and reconciliation.

1. Expressing Regret and Remorse: The core of a genuine apology lies in expressing regret and remorse. This involves acknowledging the impact of one's actions on the other person and genuinely feeling sorry for any hurt caused.

2. Taking Responsibility: A sincere apology includes taking responsibility for one's actions. It avoids deflecting blame or making excuses, demonstrating accountability and a commitment to positive change.

Strategies for Offering Genuine Apologies in Anger Management

The journey toward mastering the art of apologizing requires intentional efforts and ongoing commitment.

1. Timing and Context: Apologizing at the right time and in the appropriate context is essential. Choose a moment when both parent and child are calm and receptive to open communication.

2. Empathetic Language: Use empathetic language in your apology. Acknowledge the emotional impact on the child, and express understanding of their feelings. This empathetic approach creates a foundation for healing.

Making Amends as a Restoration Process

Making amends is the active counterpart to offering an apology—it involves tangible actions that demonstrate a commitment to positive change.

1. Defining Meaningful Amends: Meaningful amends involve actions that repair the harm caused. It goes beyond verbal apologies, encompassing concrete steps that demonstrate a genuine desire to make things right.

2. Impact on Parental Well-Being: The process of making amends not only benefits the child but also contributes to the well-being of the parent. It provides a sense of agency and empowerment, fostering a positive environment for personal growth.

Strategies for Making Amends in Anger Management

The art of making amends requires thoughtful consideration and a commitment to sustained positive change.

1. Identifying Corrective Actions: Identify specific actions that demonstrate a commitment to positive change. This could involve implementing new anger management strategies, engaging in joint activities with the child, or seeking professional support.

2. Consistency in Positive Behavior: Consistency is key in making amends. Implementing positive changes consistently reinforces the sincerity of the apology and contributes to rebuilding trust over time.

Real-Time Application of Apology and Amends in Anger Management

The real-time application of apology and amends becomes pivotal during moments of potential conflict or anger.

1. Immediate Acknowledgment and Apology: When anger results in harm, offering an immediate acknowledgment and apology is crucial. Promptly recognizing the

impact of actions and expressing genuine remorse creates a foundation for healing.

2. Tangible Actions Toward Amends: In conjunction with verbal apologies, take tangible actions toward amends. These actions should align with the identified corrective measures and demonstrate a commitment to positive change.

Seeking Professional Guidance for Apology and Amends

For parents navigating persistent challenges in offering genuine apologies and making meaningful amends, seeking professional guidance can provide valuable support.

1. Family Counseling: Family counseling sessions offer a structured environment for addressing communication dynamics. Therapists can guide parents and children through the process of offering and receiving apologies, as well as implementing effective amends.

2. Parenting Workshops: Participate in parenting workshops or support groups. These settings often include role-playing exercises, practical tools, and shared experiences that contribute to enhanced communication skills and effective amends.

The Long-Term Impact of Apology and Amends

The mastery of offering genuine apologies and making meaningful amends is a gift that reverberates through the generations—a legacy of emotional intelligence, understanding, and harmonious relationships.

1. Building Emotional Resilience in Children: Parents who navigate the journey of apology and amends contribute significantly to the emotional resilience of their children. This legacy equips the younger generation with the tools to navigate conflicts, express themselves

effectively, and cultivate healthy relationships.

2. Fostering a Culture of Emotional Accountability: A family rooted in the practice of offering genuine apologies and making meaningful amends becomes a beacon of emotional accountability. As parents model humility, responsibility, and the capacity for positive change, they cultivate a culture where conflicts are opportunities for growth, and relationships are strengthened through the transformative power of healing words and actions.

In the intricate tapestry of parenthood, offering genuine apologies and making meaningful amends emerge as threads of restoration—a testament to the resilience of familial bonds. By mastering the art of apology and amends after moments of anger, parents not only enhance their own well-being but also weave a legacy of understanding, empathy, and connection that endures through the ebbs and flows of family life. In the intentional steps of apology and amends, parents find the power to transform conflict into growth, anger into healing, and fractured connections into resilient bonds that withstand the tests of time.

6.1.2 Rebuilding Connections with Children

In the intricate dance of parenthood, where emotions often collide and conflicts arise, the art of rebuilding connections with children emerges as a profound and transformative practice—an essential skill in the pursuit of anger management mastery. This chapter explores the significance of reconnecting, unveiling how parents can navigate the aftermath of anger, foster understanding, and cultivate a resilient and harmonious family environment.

The Essence of Rebuilding Connections

The parent-child relationship is resilient, capable of weathering storms and finding renewal in the wake of conflicts. Rebuilding connections is an intentional process that involves nurturing understanding, fostering communication, and creating an environment where trust and love can flourish.

1. Defining Connection Rebuilding: Rebuilding connections involves deliberate actions aimed at repairing any ruptures in the parent-child relationship caused by anger or conflicts. It requires a commitment to understanding, empathy, and positive change.

2. Impact on Parental Well-Being: The state of connection within the parent-child relationship directly influences parental well-being. Rebuilding connections not only fosters a sense of fulfillment and joy but also contributes to a harmonious family dynamic.

Dynamics of Connection and Anger

Understanding how connection dynamics intersect with anger is essential for parents seeking mastery over their emotional responses.

1. Impact of Anger on Connection: Uncontrolled anger can strain the parent-child connection. Children may perceive anger as a threat to their emotional safety, leading to a temporary breakdown in the connection.

2. Connection Rebuilding as a Healing Journey: Rebuilding connections is a healing journey. It involves acknowledging the impact of anger, creating a safe space for communication, and taking intentional steps to restore trust and understanding.

Core Elements of Connection Rebuilding

Rebuilding connections is a nuanced process that involves specific elements aimed at fostering healing and renewal.

1. Open and Honest Communication: The foundation of connection rebuilding lies in open and honest communication. Parents should create an environment where children feel safe expressing their feelings and concerns without fear of judgment.

2. Demonstrating Empathy: Empathy is a cornerstone of connection rebuilding. Parents should strive to understand the child's perspective, acknowledge their feelings, and convey a genuine sense of care and concern.

Strategies for Rebuilding Connections in Anger Management

The journey toward mastering the art of rebuilding connections requires intentional efforts and a commitment to sustained positive change.

1. Initiating Heart-to-Heart Conversations: Heart-to-heart conversations create opportunities for connection rebuilding. Initiate discussions where both parent and child can express their feelings, share perspectives, and work towards understanding.

2. Quality Time and Shared Activities: Spending quality time and engaging in shared activities contribute to connection rebuilding. Positive experiences create lasting memories and reinforce the bond between parent and child.

Real-Time Application of Connection Rebuilding in Anger Management

The real-time application of connection rebuilding becomes pivotal during moments of potential conflict or anger.

1. Initiating Apologies and Amends: Offering genuine apologies and making meaningful amends are integral to connection rebuilding. These actions signal a commitment to positive change and contribute to healing emotional wounds.

2. Affirming Love and Support: Affirming love and support through both words and actions is crucial. Reassure the child of unconditional love, emphasizing that conflicts do not diminish the depth of the parent-child bond.

Seeking Professional Guidance for Connection Rebuilding

For parents facing persistent challenges in rebuilding connections, seeking professional guidance can provide valuable support.

1. Family Counseling: Family counseling sessions offer a structured environment for addressing communication dynamics. Therapists can guide parents and children through the process of connection rebuilding, fostering open communication and understanding.

2. Parenting Workshops: Participate in parenting workshops or support groups. These settings often provide practical tools and strategies for effective connection rebuilding within the parent-child relationship.

The Long-Term Impact of Connection Rebuilding

The mastery of connection rebuilding is a gift that echoes through the generations—a legacy of understanding, empathy, and harmonious relationships.

1. Building Resilient Family Bonds: Parents who navigate the journey of connection rebuilding contribute significantly to building resilient family bonds. This legacy equips the younger generation with the tools to navigate conflicts, express themselves effectively, and cultivate healthy relationships.

2. Fostering Emotional Intelligence in Children: A family rooted in connection rebuilding becomes a nurturing ground for emotional intelligence. As parents model effective communication, empathy, and the capacity for renewal, they foster emotional resilience and intelligence in their children.
In the rich tapestry of parenthood, rebuilding connections with children emerges as a thread of renewal—a testament to the enduring strength of familial bonds. By mastering the art of connection rebuilding after moments of anger, parents not only enhance their own well-being but also weave a legacy of understanding, empathy, and connection that resonates through the

family tapestry. In the intentional steps of connection rebuilding, parents find the power to transform conflicts into opportunities for growth, anger into healing, and fractured connections into resilient bonds that withstand the tests of time.

6.2 Strengthening Bond Through Positive Reinforcement

In the intricate dance of parenthood, where emotions sway and conflicts may arise, the art of positive reinforcement emerges as a transformative force—an essential skill in the pursuit of anger management mastery. This chapter delves into the significance of using positive reinforcement to strengthen bonds with children, revealing how parents can navigate the complexities of anger, foster understanding, and cultivate a resilient and harmonious family environment.

Embracing the Impact of Positivity in Parenting

Positivity is a catalyst for growth, healing, and connection within the parent-child relationship. Positive reinforcement involves intentionally acknowledging and rewarding positive behavior, creating an environment where love and understanding can flourish.

1. Defining Positive Reinforcement: Positive reinforcement entails the intentional use of rewards, praise, or affirmations to reinforce positive behavior. It is a proactive approach that focuses on strengths, nurturing a supportive and encouraging family dynamic.

2. Impact on Parental Well-Being: The incorporation of positive reinforcement directly influences parental well-being. It fosters a sense of accomplishment, joy, and fulfillment, contributing to a positive outlook on parenting.

Dynamics of Positivity and Anger

Understanding how positivity dynamics intersect with anger is crucial for parents seeking mastery over their emotional responses.

1. Positivity as a Counterbalance to Anger: Positive reinforcement serves as a counterbalance to anger. By intentionally highlighting and celebrating positive behaviors, parents create a foundation for open communication and connection, mitigating the impact of anger.

2. Positivity as a Preventive Measure: Positivity acts as a preventive measure against the escalation of anger. When children experience consistent positive reinforcement, they are more likely to feel secure, valued, and less prone to engage in behaviors that may trigger parental anger.

Core Elements of Positive Reinforcement

Positive reinforcement is a nuanced practice that involves specific elements aimed at fostering growth and connection.

1. Timely Acknowledgment: Timely acknowledgment is crucial in positive reinforcement. Parents should promptly recognize and affirm positive behaviors, creating a direct association between the behavior and the positive acknowledgment.

2. Authentic and Specific Praise: Authentic and specific praise enhances the impact of positive reinforcement. Rather than generic praise, parents should articulate what specific behavior or effort is being commended, reinforcing a clear connection between actions and positive acknowledgment.

Strategies for Positive Reinforcement in Anger Management

The journey toward mastering positive reinforcement requires intentional efforts and a commitment to sustained positive change.

1. Creating a Positive Reinforcement Plan: Develop a positive reinforcement plan that identifies specific behaviors to reinforce and the corresponding rewards or affirmations. This plan serves as a proactive guide for incorporating positivity into the parenting dynamic.

2. Consistent Application of Positive Language: Consistent use of positive language contributes to a nurturing environment. Parents should focus on framing communication in a positive light, emphasizing encouragement and affirmation.

Real-Time Application of Positive Reinforcement in Anger Management

The real-time application of positive reinforcement becomes pivotal during moments of potential conflict or anger.

1. Identifying Opportunities for Positivity: Actively seek opportunities for positive

reinforcement. During moments of potential conflict, intentionally look for positive behaviors to acknowledge, redirecting the focus from negative aspects to constructive actions.

2. Celebrating Small Achievements: Celebrate small achievements with enthusiasm. Recognizing even minor positive behaviors contributes to a culture of encouragement, reinforcing the notion that effort and growth are valued.

Seeking Professional Guidance for Positive Reinforcement

For parents navigating persistent challenges in incorporating positive reinforcement, seeking professional guidance can provide valuable support.

1. Parenting Workshops: Participate in parenting workshops or support groups that focus on positive reinforcement techniques. These settings often offer practical tools,

insights, and shared experiences that contribute to effective implementation.

2. Behavioral Therapy for Children: In cases where children may exhibit challenging behaviors, consider behavioral therapy. Behavioral therapists can work with parents to develop personalized positive reinforcement strategies that address specific challenges.

The Long-Term Impact of Positive Reinforcement

The mastery of positive reinforcement is a gift that resonates through the generations—a legacy of encouragement, understanding, and harmonious relationships.

1. Building Confidence and Self-Esteem in Children: Parents who embrace positive reinforcement significantly contribute to building confidence and self-esteem in their children. This legacy equips the younger

generation with the tools to navigate challenges, value their efforts, and cultivate a positive self-image.

2. Fostering a Culture of Encouragement: A family rooted in positive reinforcement becomes a culture of encouragement. As parents consistently reinforce positive behaviors, they foster an environment where children feel supported, valued, and motivated to engage in positive actions.

In the intricate tapestry of parenthood, positive reinforcement emerges as a thread of connection—a testament to the transformative power of encouragement. By mastering the art of positive reinforcement after moments of anger, parents not only enhance their own well-being but also weave a legacy of understanding, empathy, and connection that resonates through the family tapestry. In the intentional steps of positive reinforcement, parents find the power to transform conflicts into opportunities for growth, anger into constructive change, and family dynamics into a symphony of harmonious relationships that endures through the ebbs and flows of family life.

6.2.1 Encouragement and Support

In the intricate dance of parenthood, where emotions ebb and flow, the twin forces of encouragement and support emerge as transformative pillars—an indispensable duo in the pursuit of anger management mastery. This chapter explores the profound significance of providing encouragement and support, revealing how parents can navigate the complexities of anger, foster understanding, and cultivate a resilient and harmonious family environment.

The Dynamic Impact of Encouragement and Support in Parenting

Encouragement and support are catalysts for growth, emotional well-being, and the cultivation of strong bonds within the parent-child relationship. They create an environment where children feel valued, supported, and empowered to navigate the challenges of life.

1. Defining Encouragement: Encouragement involves offering words, gestures, or actions that inspire and uplift. It is a deliberate expression of belief in a child's abilities and potential, fostering a positive outlook and a sense of self-efficacy.

2. The Essence of Support: Support encompasses the provision of assistance, understanding, and a nurturing presence. It involves standing by a child during both triumphs and challenges, creating a secure foundation for emotional well-being.

Impact on Parental Well-Being

The incorporation of encouragement and support directly influences parental well-being, contributing to a sense of fulfillment, purpose, and joy in the parenting journey. By uplifting their children, parents also experience the profound satisfaction of nurturing their development and resilience.

Dynamics of Encouragement, Support, and Anger

Understanding how encouragement and support intersect with anger is crucial for parents seeking mastery over their emotional responses.

1. Mitigating the Impact of Anger: Encouragement and support act as buffers against the impact of anger. When children feel encouraged and supported, the emotional fallout of anger is mitigated, fostering resilience and a sense of emotional safety.

2. Transforming Negative Dynamics: By infusing positive elements into the parent-child relationship through encouragement and support, parents can transform negative dynamics associated with anger. This transformation opens avenues

for understanding, communication, and growth.

Core Elements of Encouragement and Support

Encouragement and support are nuanced practices that involve specific elements aimed at fostering growth, resilience, and connection.

1. Affirmative Communication: Affirmative communication involves using positive language to convey belief in a child's abilities. It includes verbal affirmations, compliments, and expressions of pride and confidence.

2. Active Presence and Listening: Active presence and listening form the foundation of support. Being fully present and attentive to a child's thoughts and feelings communicates a sense of understanding and validation.

Strategies for Providing Encouragement and Support in Anger Management

The journey toward mastering the art of encouragement and support requires intentional efforts and a commitment to sustained positive change.

1. Daily Affirmations and Acknowledgments: Incorporate daily affirmations and acknowledgments into your interactions. Take moments to highlight specific achievements, efforts, or positive behaviors, reinforcing the child's sense of value.

2. Creating a Safe Space for Expression:
Foster an environment where children feel safe expressing their thoughts and emotions. By creating a non-judgmental space, parents encourage open communication and strengthen the parent-child bond.

Real-Time Application of Encouragement and Support in Anger Management

The real-time application of encouragement and support becomes pivotal during moments of potential conflict or anger.

1. Immediate Affirmation of Effort: In moments where challenges arise or conflicts occur, immediately affirm the child's effort. Acknowledge their attempts, emphasize the learning process, and provide reassurance that mistakes are opportunities for growth.

2. Expressing Unconditional Love: Express unconditional love consistently. Reinforce the idea that a parent's love is unwavering, even in the face of anger or conflicts. This reassurance creates a stable foundation for emotional security.

Seeking Professional Guidance for Encouragement and Support

For parents facing persistent challenges in providing encouragement and support, seeking professional guidance can offer valuable insights.

1. Parenting Seminars and Workshops: Participate in parenting seminars or workshops that focus on positive parenting techniques. These settings often provide practical tools, role-playing exercises, and expert guidance on incorporating encouragement and support into daily interactions.

2. Therapeutic Support: In cases where persistent challenges or underlying issues contribute to anger, consider seeking therapeutic support. Professional therapists can work with parents to develop personalized strategies for fostering encouragement and support within the family dynamic.

The Long-Term Impact of Encouragement and Support

The mastery of providing encouragement and support is a gift that reverberates through the generations—a legacy of resilience, confidence, and harmonious relationships.

1. Building Confidence and Self-Esteem in Children: Parents who consistently provide encouragement and support significantly contribute to building confidence and self-esteem in their children. This legacy equips the younger generation with the tools to navigate challenges, believe in their abilities, and cultivate a positive self-image.

2. Fostering Emotional Resilience: A family rooted in encouragement and support becomes a nurturing ground for emotional resilience. As parents model positive communication, understanding, and unwavering support, they foster emotional intelligence and resilience in their children.

In the intricate tapestry of parenthood, encouragement and support emerge as threads of empowerment—a testament to the transformative power of positive influence. By mastering the art of encouragement and support after moments of anger, parents not only enhance their own well-being but also weave a legacy of understanding, empathy, and connection that resonates through the family tapestry. In the intentional steps of encouragement and support, parents find the power to transform conflicts into opportunities for growth, anger into constructive change, and family dynamics into a symphony of harmonious relationships that endures through the ebbs and flows of family life.

6.2.2 Creating a Positive Home Environment

In the intricate tapestry of parenthood, the environment within the home acts as a canvas upon which the colors of family life are painted. This chapter delves into the profound significance of creating a positive home environment—a sanctuary where children can thrive, conflicts find resolution, and the art of anger management is masterfully practiced.

The Essence of a Positive Home Environment

A positive home environment is more than just physical surroundings; it's a dynamic atmosphere shaped by emotions, communication, and the overall well-being of its occupants. It is a space where love, understanding, and support lay the foundation for healthy family dynamics.

1. Defining a Positive Home Environment: A positive home environment is characterized by warmth, open communication, and a sense of security. It nurtures emotional well-being, encourages positive interactions, and provides a backdrop for the practice of effective anger management.

2. Impact on Parental Well-Being: The creation of a positive home environment directly influences parental well-being. It fosters a sense of joy, satisfaction, and purpose, contributing to a harmonious and fulfilling family life.

Dynamics of a Positive Home Environment and Anger

Understanding how the dynamics of a positive home environment intersect with anger is crucial for parents seeking mastery over their emotional responses.

1. Buffering Against the Impact of Anger: A positive home environment acts as a buffer against the impact of anger. When children and parents experience the support, understanding, and positivity within their home, conflicts are approached with greater resilience and emotional intelligence.

2. Fostering Healthy Communication: Open communication is a hallmark of a positive home environment. When family members feel comfortable expressing their thoughts and feelings, the potential for misunderstandings that lead to anger diminishes.

Core Elements of a Positive Home Environment

Cultivating a positive home environment involves intentional efforts and a commitment to nurturing emotional well-being.

1. Clear Communication Channels: Clear and open communication channels create an environment where family members feel heard and understood. Encouraging dialogue fosters an atmosphere where conflicts can be addressed constructively.

2. Shared Values and Expectations: Establishing shared values and expectations

within the family provides a framework for positive behavior. When everyone understands the collective vision for the home, it promotes unity and reduces the likelihood of conflicts leading to anger.

Strategies for Creating a Positive Home Environment in Anger Management

The journey toward mastering the creation of a positive home environment requires intentional efforts and a commitment to sustained positive change.

1. Family Meetings and Check-Ins: Regular family meetings provide a platform for open communication. Use these gatherings to discuss concerns, express appreciation, and collaboratively establish guidelines for maintaining a positive home environment.

2. Designated Safe Spaces: Create designated safe spaces within the home where family members can retreat to when emotions run high. These spaces serve as

sanctuaries for emotional release, reflection, and the practice of calming techniques.

Real-Time Application of a Positive Home Environment in Anger Management

The real-time application of a positive home environment becomes pivotal during moments of potential conflict or anger.

1. Modeling Positive Behavior: Parents play a pivotal role in modeling positive behavior. By exemplifying effective anger management and demonstrating kindness, they create a template for children to follow, contributing to a harmonious family atmosphere.

2. Celebrating Achievements, Big and Small: Actively celebrate achievements, both big and small. This fosters an environment where effort and growth are acknowledged and valued, reducing the likelihood of anger stemming from feelings of inadequacy.

Seeking Professional Guidance for a Positive Home Environment

For parents navigating persistent challenges in creating a positive home environment, seeking professional guidance can provide valuable support.

1. Family Therapy Sessions: Family therapy sessions offer a structured environment for addressing communication dynamics. Therapists can guide parents and children in the process of creating a positive home environment, fostering open communication and understanding.

2. Parenting Workshops: Participate in parenting workshops or support groups. These settings often provide practical tools, insights, and shared experiences that contribute to effective home environment cultivation.

The Long-Term Impact of a Positive Home Environment

The mastery of creating a positive home environment is a gift that echoes through the generations—a legacy of love, understanding, and harmonious relationships.

1. Building Emotional Resilience in Children: Children raised in a positive home environment develop emotional resilience. This legacy equips the younger generation with the tools to navigate challenges, express themselves effectively, and cultivate healthy relationships.

2. Fostering a Culture of Positivity: A family rooted in a positive home environment becomes a culture of positivity. As parents consistently model positive behavior and communication, they foster an environment where conflicts are opportunities for growth, and relationships are strengthened through

the transformative power of love, understanding, and harmony.

In the intricate tapestry of parenthood, the creation of a positive home environment emerges as a thread of harmony—a testament to the transformative power of intentional living. By mastering the art of cultivating positivity within their homes after moments of anger, parents not only enhance their own well-being but also weave a legacy of understanding, empathy, and connection that resonates through the family tapestry. In the intentional steps of creating a positive home environment, parents find the power to transform conflicts into opportunities for growth, anger into constructive change, and family life into a symphony of harmonious relationships that endures through the ebbs and flows of daily living.

Chapter 7: Seeking Professional Help

7.1 When to Consider Therapy

In the intricate journey of parenthood, the waves of emotions can sometimes become tumultuous, leading to moments of anger and frustration. While mastering self-control is an essential aspect, there are instances where seeking therapy becomes a valuable and transformative choice. This chapter explores the nuanced considerations of when to consider therapy for parents aiming to master anger management, offering insights into the signs, benefits, and the profound impact therapy can have on the path to emotional well-being.

Recognizing Signs That Therapy May Be Beneficial

Parental anger, when unaddressed, can create challenges that extend beyond personal well-being and impact the entire family dynamic. Recognizing the signs that therapy may be beneficial is a proactive step toward fostering positive change.

1. Consistent Struggles with Anger: If anger becomes a consistent challenge, erupting frequently and intensely, it may indicate an underlying issue that could benefit from therapeutic exploration.

2. Impact on Relationships: When anger starts to strain relationships within the family—whether it's with a partner, children, or other family members—it's a clear indicator that therapeutic intervention may be helpful.

3. Negative Effects on Parental Well-Being: If anger negatively impacts parental well-being, leading to feelings of guilt, shame, or a sense of loss of control, therapy can provide a supportive space for understanding and coping with these emotions.

The Benefits of Therapy for Anger Management

Therapy offers a structured and supportive environment for parents to explore the root causes of their anger, develop coping strategies, and foster positive change. Here are some key benefits:

1. Understanding Triggers: Therapy helps parents identify the underlying triggers of their anger. This self-awareness is crucial for developing effective coping mechanisms and preventive strategies.

2. Learning Coping Strategies: Therapists provide tools and coping strategies tailored to the individual, helping parents navigate moments of anger with resilience and emotional intelligence.

3. Improving Communication Skills: Therapy often involves improving communication skills, helping parents express their emotions constructively and

fostering healthier interactions within the family.

4. Enhancing Emotional Regulation: Through therapeutic techniques, parents can enhance their emotional regulation, gaining the ability to manage stress and frustration more effectively.

When to Consider Therapy: Practical Considerations

While recognizing the emotional signs is crucial, practical considerations also play a role in deciding when therapy may be beneficial for anger management mastery.

1. Persistent Challenges Despite Efforts: If despite personal efforts and lifestyle changes, anger management challenges persist, therapy can provide additional tools and perspectives.

2. Impact on Parenting Effectiveness: When anger interferes with effective parenting,

impacting a parent's ability to provide a nurturing and supportive environment, therapy becomes an essential consideration.

3. Feedback from Loved Ones: Insightful feedback from loved ones can be a valuable indicator. If family members express concern about a parent's anger, it may be time to consider therapy for the benefit of the entire family.

Types of Therapy for Anger Management

Several therapeutic approaches can be effective in addressing anger management issues. The choice of therapy depends on individual preferences, needs, and the therapist's expertise. Some common types include:

1. Cognitive-Behavioral Therapy (CBT): CBT focuses on identifying and changing negative thought patterns and behaviors. It is particularly effective in addressing the cognitive aspects of anger.

2. Mindfulness-Based Approaches: Mindfulness techniques can help parents stay present in the moment, fostering emotional regulation and reducing impulsive reactions.

3. Family Therapy: Family therapy involves addressing anger within the context of family dynamics. It can be beneficial in improving communication and understanding among family members.

Overcoming Stigma and Seeking Support

The decision to pursue therapy is often hindered by the stigma surrounding mental health. However, overcoming this stigma is a crucial step toward seeking the support needed for effective anger management.

1. Shifting Perspectives: Viewing therapy as a proactive and empowering step toward personal growth can shift perspectives and reduce the stigma associated with seeking professional support.

2. Normalizing Mental Health Care: Normalizing mental health care within the family and society at large creates an environment where seeking therapy for anger management is seen as a positive and proactive choice.

Realizing the Long-Term Impact

The long-term impact of therapy for anger management extends beyond personal well-being. It contributes to the creation of a healthier family environment and sets the stage for positive generational change.

1. Building Resilient Family Bonds: Through therapy, parents can build resilient family bonds by addressing anger issues at their roots and fostering healthier communication and understanding.

2. Cultivating Emotional Intelligence in Children: As parents model self-awareness and emotional regulation, they contribute to the emotional intelligence of their children,

equipping them with essential skills for navigating their own emotions.

In the rich tapestry of parenthood, the decision to consider therapy for anger management is an empowering choice—a testament to the commitment to personal growth and the well-being of the entire family. By recognizing the signs, understanding the benefits, and overcoming stigma, parents embark on a transformative journey that extends beyond the mastery of anger to the creation of a harmonious and resilient family environment. In the intentional steps of therapy, parents find the power to transform conflicts into opportunities for growth, anger into constructive change, and family dynamics into a symphony of harmonious relationships that endures through the ebbs and flows of family life.

7.1.1 Signs that Professional Help is Needed

Parenting is a complex journey marked by a spectrum of emotions, and anger can sometimes emerge as a formidable challenge. While mastering anger management is a goal for many parents, there are moments when recognizing the need for professional help becomes a crucial step toward sustainable well-being. This chapter explores the nuanced signs that indicate professional assistance may be beneficial, offering insights into the complexities of anger management and the transformative impact of seeking expert guidance.

The Uncharted Terrain of Parental Anger

Parental anger, when left unaddressed, can permeate various aspects of family life, impacting relationships, communication, and overall well-being. Recognizing the signs that professional help is needed involves navigating the uncharted terrain where personal challenges intersect with the complexities of parenting.

1. Intense and Frequent Outbursts: If anger manifests as intense and frequent outbursts, extending beyond occasional moments of frustration, it may indicate a deeper issue that requires professional exploration.

2. Impact on Family Relationships: When anger significantly impacts family relationships, creating strained dynamics or a hostile environment, seeking professional help becomes a proactive step toward restoring harmony.

3. Feelings of Guilt and Helplessness: Persistent feelings of guilt, helplessness, or an inability to control anger can be indicators that underlying issues may benefit from the specialized support provided by mental health professionals.

The Complex Interplay of Emotions

Parental anger is often entwined with a complex interplay of emotions, ranging from stress and frustration to deeper-seated issues such as unresolved trauma or unmet needs. Recognizing these emotional intricacies is a pivotal step in understanding the signs that professional help may be necessary.

1. Escalation Despite Efforts: If efforts to manage anger prove ineffective and conflicts consistently escalate, it suggests that the emotional roots of anger may require exploration in a therapeutic setting.

2. Difficulty Identifying Triggers: Difficulty in identifying the triggers of anger or understanding the underlying emotions driving the anger may indicate the need for professional guidance to delve into the subconscious aspects of emotional responses.

Impact on Parental Well-Being

The well-being of parents is intricately connected to effective anger management. Recognizing the signs that anger is significantly impacting personal well-being is a critical aspect of understanding when professional help is warranted.

1. Negative Effects on Mental Health: If anger is contributing to negative effects on mental health, such as increased stress, anxiety, or a sense of emotional exhaustion, it signals the importance of seeking professional intervention.

2. Strained Physical Health: Persistent anger can manifest in physical health issues, such as elevated blood pressure or chronic tension. Recognizing these physical signs underscores the holistic impact of anger on overall well-being.

Behavioral Patterns and Outcomes

Observing behavioral patterns and the outcomes of anger is essential in gauging whether professional help is necessary. Identifying patterns that persist despite personal efforts highlights the need for specialized support.

1. Repetitive Destructive Behaviors: If anger consistently leads to destructive behaviors, whether verbal or physical, seeking professional help is imperative to break these patterns and develop healthier coping mechanisms.

2. Impact on Parenting Effectiveness: When anger interferes with effective parenting, hindering the ability to provide a nurturing and supportive environment, it emphasizes the necessity of professional guidance to enhance parenting skills.

External Feedback and Perspectives

External feedback from loved ones, friends, or colleagues can serve as valuable indicators. If those in close relationships express concern about a parent's anger or well-being, it may be time to consider professional help.

1. Expressions of Concern from Family: If family members express worry or discomfort about a parent's anger, it signifies the broader impact on the family dynamic and underscores the importance of seeking professional assistance.

2. Workplace or Social Feedback: Feedback from the workplace or social circles that suggests difficulty managing anger in various contexts is a compelling signal that seeking professional help may lead to positive change.

Overcoming Stigma and Accepting Support

One of the barriers to seeking professional help for anger management is the stigma surrounding mental health. Overcoming this stigma involves recognizing the value of seeking support and understanding that it is a proactive step toward personal growth.

1. Viewing Therapy as a Strength: Shifting perspectives to view therapy as a strength rather than a weakness reframes the narrative around seeking professional help and encourages a more positive and open approach to mental health.

2. Normalizing Mental Health Conversations: Normalizing conversations about mental health within the family and society helps create an environment where seeking professional help for anger management is seen as a natural and beneficial choice.

When to Consider Professional Help: A Holistic Approach

Making The decision to seek professional help for anger management is a complex and personal choice. A holistic approach involves considering emotional, relational, and well-being aspects to determine when the time is right for therapeutic intervention.

1. Exhaustion of Personal Resources: When personal efforts and resources to manage anger are exhausted, seeking professional help becomes a logical and proactive step toward accessing additional tools and support.

2. Commitment to Personal Growth: A commitment to personal growth and the well-being of the family underscores the transformative potential of therapy for anger management. It signifies an intentional choice to break patterns and cultivate positive change.

Types of Therapy for Anger Management

Various therapeutic modalities can effectively address anger management issues. From cognitive-behavioral therapy (CBT) to anger management counseling, the choice of therapy depends on individual needs, preferences, and the expertise of the therapist.

1. Cognitive-Behavioral Therapy (CBT): CBT is a widely used approach that focuses on identifying and changing negative thought patterns and behaviors associated with anger, offering practical tools for emotional regulation.

2. Individual or Group Counseling: Individual or group counseling provides a supportive environment for exploring the roots of anger, developing coping strategies, and sharing experiences with others facing similar challenges.

The Transformative Impact of Seeking Help

Recognizing the signs that professional help is needed is a powerful step toward transformative change. Seeking support for anger management is an investment in personal well-being and the creation of a healthier family environment.

1. Breaking Generational Patterns: Therapy has the potential to break generational patterns of anger and contribute to positive change that resonates through family dynamics, fostering healthy relationships for generations to come.

2. Enhancing Self-Awareness: Professional help enhances self-awareness, allowing parents to gain insights into the root causes of their anger and empowering them to make informed choices for personal growth.

In the intricate landscape of parenting, recognizing the signs that professional help is needed for anger management mastery is a courageous step toward emotional well-being. By understanding the nuanced indicators, overcoming stigma, and accepting support, parents embark on a transformative journey that extends beyond personal growth to the creation of a harmonious and resilient family environment. In the intentional steps of seeking professional help, parents find the power to transform conflicts into opportunities for growth, anger into constructive change, and family dynamics into a symphony of harmonious relationships that endures through the ebbs and flows of family life.

7.1.2 Types of Therapeutic Approaches

The journey toward mastering anger management is a nuanced and individualized process, and therapeutic approaches play a pivotal role in guiding parents toward transformative change. This chapter delves into the diverse landscape of therapeutic interventions, offering an in-depth exploration of various approaches designed to empower parents in their quest to be the masters of their emotions.

1. Cognitive-Behavioral Therapy (CBT): Cognitive-Behavioral Therapy (CBT) stands as a cornerstone in the realm of anger management. This approach targets the interplay between thoughts, emotions, and behaviors, aiming to identify and alter negative patterns. In CBT, parents work collaboratively with therapists to recognize distorted thought patterns contributing to anger, challenge them, and replace them with more constructive alternatives. By honing in on the cognitive aspects of anger, CBT equips parents with practical tools to reframe perceptions, regulate emotions, and foster healthier behavioral responses.

2. Mindfulness-Based Approaches: Mindfulness-based approaches draw

inspiration from ancient contemplative practices, placing a strong emphasis on present-moment awareness. Mindfulness techniques, such as meditation and deep-breathing exercises, enable parents to cultivate a heightened sense of awareness and observe their thoughts and emotions without judgment. This heightened awareness becomes a powerful tool in recognizing the early signs of anger, providing a pause for reflection and promoting intentional, measured responses. By integrating mindfulness into their lives, parents embark on a journey of self-discovery, enhancing emotional regulation and resilience.

3. Dialectical Behavior Therapy (DBT): Dialectical Behavior Therapy (DBT) is a comprehensive approach that harmonizes acceptance and change strategies. Originally developed for individuals with borderline personality disorder, DBT has proven effective in addressing anger and emotional dysregulation. DBT introduces skills for

distress tolerance, emotion regulation, and interpersonal effectiveness. In the context of anger management, DBT encourages parents to accept their emotions without judgment while simultaneously working toward constructive changes. The synthesis of acceptance and change empowers parents to navigate the complexities of anger with a balanced and holistic perspective.

4.   Psychodynamic   Therapy: Psychodynamic therapy delves into the realm of unconscious influences, exploring how past experiences shape present emotions and behaviors. By unraveling the layers of unconscious thoughts and emotions, parents gain insights into the roots of their anger. Psychodynamic therapy often involves exploring early life experiences, relationships, and unresolved issues that may contribute to emotional responses. As parents gain awareness of these influences, they can work toward resolving underlying conflicts and forging a path toward healthier emotional responses.

5. Family Therapy: Anger within a family context necessitates a therapeutic approach that considers the dynamics of the entire familial unit. Family therapy is designed to address relational patterns and communication styles that contribute to anger. In a safe and supportive environment, family members, including parents and children, collaborate with a therapist to enhance understanding, improve communication, and cultivate a harmonious family environment. By involving all family members in the therapeutic process, family therapy acknowledges the interconnectedness of emotions and relationships, fostering collective growth and resilience.

6. Solution-Focused Brief Therapy (SFBT): Solution-Focused Brief Therapy (SFBT) is grounded in the belief that solutions can be identified and implemented swiftly. Instead of delving extensively into the origins of problems, SFBT focuses on identifying

goals and practical steps toward achieving them. In the context of anger management, SFBT assists parents in envisioning a future where anger is effectively managed, and then collaboratively develops strategies to make that vision a reality. By concentrating on solutions rather than dwelling on problems, SFBT empowers parents to enact positive change in a time-efficient manner.

7. Gestalt Therapy: Gestalt therapy invites individuals to fully engage with their present experiences and emotions. This approach emphasizes the importance of awareness, personal responsibility, and the integration of fragmented aspects of the self. In the context of anger management, Gestalt therapy encourages parents to explore the full spectrum of their emotions, fostering a holistic understanding of anger and its underlying causes. Through techniques such as role-playing and guided dialogues, parents gain clarity on the present moment, paving the way for self-acceptance and intentional emotional responses.

8. Narrative Therapy: Narrative therapy views individuals as the authors of their own stories and seeks to rewrite narratives that contribute to distress. In the context of anger management, this approach involves exploring the stories parents tell themselves about their anger and reframing them in a more empowering light. By externalizing the problem and separating it from one's identity, parents can construct alternative narratives that emphasize resilience, growth, and the capacity for change. Narrative therapy offers a creative and empowering lens through which parents can reimagine their relationship with anger.

Selecting the Right Therapeutic Approach

Choosing the most fitting therapeutic approach is a highly individualized process that considers the unique needs, preferences, and circumstances of each parent. The effectiveness of a therapeutic approach hinges on the collaborative relationship between the parent and therapist, emphasizing trust, open communication, and a shared commitment to the journey of anger management mastery.

In the rich tapestry of anger management, the diverse array of therapeutic approaches provides a mosaic of possibilities for parents seeking mastery over their emotions. By exploring these avenues—whether through cognitive restructuring, mindfulness cultivation, or family dynamics enhancement—parents embark on a transformative journey that goes beyond symptom alleviation to the profound rewiring of emotional responses. In the intentional steps of therapeutic exploration, parents find the power to transform conflicts into opportunities for growth, anger into constructive change, and family dynamics into a symphony of harmonious relationships that endures through the ebbs and flows of family life.

7.2 Involving Family Members in the Healing Process

The intricate dance of familial relationships often encounters moments of discord, and anger can emerge as a powerful force that shapes the dynamics within a family. In the pursuit of mastering anger management, involving family members in the healing process becomes a transformative endeavor. This chapter explores the profound impact of including the family unit in the journey toward emotional mastery, fostering understanding, communication, and harmonious relationships.

Understanding the Family as a System

Family dynamics are akin to an intricate ecosystem where each member contributes to the overall balance. In the context of anger management, acknowledging the interconnectedness of family members and their emotions is a fundamental aspect of initiating healing. Rather than viewing anger as an isolated individual experience, involving family members recognizes it as a shared journey, inviting collective growth and resilience.

The Ripple Effect of Anger in the Family

Anger, when unaddressed, can create a ripple effect that touches every corner of family life. It permeates communication, strains relationships, and influences the emotional well-being of each family member. Recognizing the far-reaching impact of anger underscores the importance of involving the entire family in the healing process.

Building a Foundation of Open Communication

Effective communication lies at the heart of any thriving family. In the context of anger management, involving family members necessitates the establishment of a foundation where open and honest communication can flourish. Creating a safe space for family members to express their thoughts, feelings, and concerns fosters a supportive environment that is conducive to healing.

Family Meetings

Family meetings serve as a structured and collaborative forum for expression. These gatherings provide an opportunity for each family member, including parents and children, to share their perspectives on how anger affects them. By fostering an atmosphere of mutual respect and active listening, family meetings become a space where emotions can be acknowledged, and collective solutions can be explored.

Parental Transparency

Parents play a pivotal role in modeling emotional regulation for their children.

Involving family members in the healing process begins with parental transparency—openly acknowledging personal struggles with anger and demonstrating a commitment to positive change. By doing so, parents provide a powerful example that encourages children to navigate their own emotions with resilience and self-awareness.

Encouraging Shared Responsibility

Healing from anger is a shared responsibility that involves every member of the family. Involving family members in setting shared goals for anger management cultivates a sense of ownership and collective commitment. Whether through establishing communication guidelines or practicing coping strategies together, shared responsibility fosters a collaborative ethos that strengthens family bonds.

Family Therapy

The inclusion of family therapy in the healing process offers a structured and guided exploration of family dynamics. Therapists trained in family systems can help identify patterns of communication, power dynamics, and unresolved issues that contribute to anger. Through the therapeutic process, family members gain insights into their roles within the family unit and work collaboratively toward creating positive change.

Developing a Family Action Plan

Involving family members in the healing process often involves developing a family action plan. This plan outlines specific strategies, communication tools, and coping mechanisms that the family agrees to implement collectively. By creating a roadmap for change, the family action plan becomes a tangible expression of the shared commitment to mastering anger and fostering harmony.

Educational Workshops

Educational workshops focused on anger management can empower the entire family with knowledge and practical skills. These workshops provide a space for learning about the roots of anger, effective communication techniques, and strategies for emotional regulation. By participating together, family members gain a shared understanding that forms the basis for mutual support.

Fostering Empathy Among Family Members

Empathy is a cornerstone of healing within the family. Involving family members in the process of anger management encourages the development of empathy—understanding and validating each other's experiences. Fostering empathy creates an emotional bridge that transcends individual perspectives, fostering a collective mindset of compassion and support.

Individual Reflection Within the Family Context

While the healing process involves the family as a whole, individual reflection within the family context is equally vital. Each family member, including parents, can engage in personal introspection to identify their triggers, emotional responses, and coping mechanisms. By sharing these reflections within the family, a deeper understanding emerges, paving the way for collaborative growth.

Celebrating Progress as a Family Achievement

As the family embarks on the journey of healing, celebrating progress becomes a shared achievement. Recognizing and acknowledging improvements in communication, emotional regulation, and overall family dynamics reinforces the collective commitment to positive change. Celebrations serve as milestones, reminding each family member of their integral role in the ongoing process of anger management mastery.

In the symphony of family life, involving family members in the healing process of parental anger management mastery is akin to orchestrating harmony. By recognizing the interconnectedness of emotions, fostering open communication, and committing to shared responsibility, families embark on a transformative journey that transcends individual struggles. In the intentional steps of involving family members, parents find the power to transform conflicts into opportunities for growth, anger into constructive change, and family dynamics into a symphony of harmonious relationships that endures through the ebbs and flows of family life.

7.2.1 Family Counseling

In the intricate dance of family life, emotions weave a profound tapestry that shapes the dynamics within the household. When anger becomes a prominent thread in this intricate fabric, family counseling emerges as a compass guiding parents toward emotional mastery. This chapter embarks on a compassionate odyssey, exploring the transformative landscape of family counseling in the context of parental anger management, fostering understanding, communication, and the harmonious orchestration of familial relationships.

The Holistic Lens of Family Counseling

Family counseling operates under the belief that the family unit is an interconnected system where the emotional experiences of one member resonate throughout. In the realm of anger management, family counseling adopts a holistic lens, acknowledging that individual expressions of anger are entwined with the dynamics of the entire family. By viewing anger through this comprehensive perspective, family counseling becomes a therapeutic avenue for collective healing.

Creating a Safe Haven for Expression

At the core of family counseling is the creation of a safe and supportive haven where family members can express their thoughts, feelings, and concerns without judgment. This nurturing environment encourages open communication and provides a space for each family member, including parents, to share their experiences with anger. Through the guidance of a skilled family therapist, the family collectively embarks on a journey of self-discovery and mutual understanding.

Navigating the Complexity of Family Dynamics

Family dynamics are a complex interplay of relationships, roles, and communication patterns. In the context of anger management, family counseling delves into the intricate layers of these dynamics, seeking to identify patterns that contribute to anger and conflict. By navigating the complexity of family interactions, a family therapist assists in unraveling the emotional threads that, when addressed, contribute to a more harmonious family tapestry.

The Therapeutic Dance of Family Meetings

Family meetings, orchestrated within the framework of family counseling, become a therapeutic dance where emotions are acknowledged, and solutions are collaboratively explored. These structured gatherings provide a designated space for each family member to share their experiences with anger, fostering a sense of unity and collective responsibility. Family meetings serve as a crucible for transformation, where conflicts are not only addressed but are opportunities for growth and understanding.

Addressing Parental Transparency in a Supportive Context

A cornerstone of family counseling is parental transparency—the willingness of parents to openly acknowledge their struggles with anger. In this supportive context, parents model vulnerability and authenticity, creating an environment where family members, especially children, feel empowered to express their own emotions. Parental transparency becomes a catalyst for trust, strengthening the therapeutic bond within the family unit.

Shared Responsibility and Collaborative Goal-Setting

Family counseling encourages the distribution of shared responsibility among family members, emphasizing that anger management is a collective journey.

Through collaborative goal-setting, the family collectively establishes aspirations and strategies for managing anger. This shared responsibility fosters a sense of unity, where every family member plays a vital role in the ongoing process of emotional mastery.

The Guiding Hand of a Family Therapist

Central to the transformative journey of family counseling is the guiding hand of a skilled family therapist. Trained in navigating the complexities of family dynamics, a family therapist serves as a mediator, facilitator, and catalyst for positive change. Through a combination of therapeutic techniques, the therapist assists the family in gaining insights, developing coping strategies, and fostering effective communication.

Encouraging Empathy and Understanding

A pivotal aspect of family counseling is the encouragement of empathy and understanding among family members. By delving into the experiences and perspectives of each family member, the therapeutic process nurtures a compassionate atmosphere. This empathy serves as a bridge that transcends individual viewpoints, fostering a collective mindset of understanding and support.

Creating Individual and Collective Action Plans

In the collaborative space of family counseling, individual and collective action plans are crafted to guide the family toward positive change. These plans outline specific strategies, communication tools, and coping mechanisms tailored to the unique needs of each family member. By creating a roadmap for emotional mastery, the family gains a tangible tool that serves as a compass in the ongoing journey of anger management.

Family counseling

Family counseling acknowledges and celebrates progress as a family-wide achievement. Recognizing milestones in communication, emotional regulation, and overall family dynamics becomes a collective celebration. These moments of acknowledgment serve as affirmations of the family's commitment to positive change, reinforcing the transformative impact of the therapeutic process.

In the symphony of family life, family counseling emerges as a conductor guiding the family toward a harmonious crescendo. By creating a safe haven for expression, addressing parental transparency, and fostering shared responsibility, family counseling becomes an odyssey of emotional mastery. In the intentional steps of involving family members through counseling, parents find the power to transform conflicts into opportunities for growth, anger into constructive change, and family dynamics into a symphony of harmonious relationships that endures through the ebbs and flows of family life.

7.2.2 Support Groups for Parents

Parenting is a journey marked by both joy and challenges, and the emotion of anger can sometimes become a formidable companion along the way. In the quest for mastering anger management, support groups for parents emerge as a transformative community—a collective sanctuary where shared experiences, mutual understanding, and the wisdom of the group guide parents toward emotional mastery. This chapter embarks on an exploration of the profound impact of support groups, illuminating the pathways toward empowerment, resilience, and the harmonious orchestration of parental emotions.

The Power of Shared Experience

Support groups are a tapestry woven with shared experiences, binding parents together through the common thread of navigating anger. In the realm of anger management, these groups provide a space where parents can express their thoughts, fears, and triumphs without judgment. The power of shared experience fosters a sense of belonging and validation, assuring parents that they are not alone in their journey.

Creating a Nurturing Community

Support groups function as nurturing communities where parents, often facing similar challenges, come together to support one another. This communal atmosphere cultivates a sense of understanding and compassion, as parents realize that their struggles with anger are not isolated incidents but part of a collective human experience. The group becomes a refuge—a place where vulnerability is met with empathy and acceptance.

Diverse Perspectives, Unified Goals

In the mosaic of a support group, diverse perspectives converge with a unity of purpose. Parents from various backgrounds, cultures, and life situations bring a rich tapestry of insights into the complexities of anger management. The shared goal of emotional mastery unifies the group, creating a collaborative ethos where diverse experiences contribute to a holistic understanding of anger.

Open Dialogue and Active Listening

Support groups thrive on open dialogue and active listening. Within the safety of the group, parents share their challenges, triumphs, and strategies for managing anger. The reciprocity of active listening creates an environment where each participant feels heard and valued. As parents articulate their experiences, they not only find solace in expression but also gain insights from the collective wisdom of the group.

Peer Support

Peer support stands as a pillar of strength within support groups. The acknowledgment that fellow parents, facing similar struggles, can offer empathetic guidance creates a supportive network. Parents learn from each other's successes and setbacks, finding inspiration and encouragement in the shared resilience of the group. This peer support becomes a lifeline, reinforcing the notion that together, parents can overcome the challenges of anger.

Guided Facilitation by Professionals

Many support groups benefit from guided facilitation by professionals skilled in anger management and group dynamics. These facilitators, often therapists or counselors, provide structure to the group discussions, offer expert insights, and guide participants in developing coping strategies. The presence of a skilled facilitator enhances the therapeutic value of the support group, ensuring that the collective journey is navigated with expertise and compassion.

Anonymous Sharing

The anonymity often offered by support groups creates a safe space for vulnerability. Parents can openly share their experiences, concerns, and strategies without fear of judgment or stigma. This anonymity fosters a climate where parents feel free to explore their emotions authentically, contributing to a genuine and open exchange within the group.

Realizing Commonality in Struggles

In the shared narrative of a support group, parents come to realize the commonality in their struggles with anger. The recognition that others face similar challenges dismantles the isolation that anger can sometimes breed. Parents understand that anger is a universal emotion and that seeking support is a strength—an acknowledgment that transcends individual differences and connects them in a shared pursuit of emotional mastery.

Group Rituals and Practices

Support groups often incorporate rituals and practices that foster a sense of unity and purpose. These may include mindfulness exercises, shared goal-setting sessions, or group affirmations. These rituals become touchstones, grounding the group in a collective commitment to positive change and emotional well-being.

Crisis Intervention and Timely Guidance

In moments of heightened distress, support groups provide a form of crisis intervention. The group becomes a source of timely guidance, offering coping strategies and reassurance. The collective wisdom of the group, combined with the expertise of facilitators, ensures that parents facing acute challenges in anger management receive the support they need in real-time.

Celebrating Milestones

Support groups celebrate milestones in the journey of anger management mastery. Whether it's a parent sharing a successful strategy, overcoming a specific challenge, or expressing newfound self-awareness, these moments become collective victories. Celebrations within the group reinforce the idea that transformation is an ongoing process, marked by shared achievements and a collective commitment to emotional well-being.

In the symphony of parenting, support groups for anger management mastery resonate as a harmonious composition of shared resilience. Through the power of shared experience, open dialogue, and peer support, parents find solace, understanding, and inspiration within the group. In the intentional steps of joining a support group, parents discover the power to transform conflicts into opportunities for growth, anger into constructive change, and the journey of parenting into a symphony of harmonious relationships that endures through the ebbs and flows of family life.

Chapter 8: Sustaining Positive Change

8.1 Creating a Long-Term Action Plan

Embarking on the journey of anger management is not a fleeting endeavor but rather a lifelong commitment to emotional well-being and harmonious relationships within the family. In this chapter, we delve into the intricacies of creating a comprehensive and long-term action plan, providing parents with a roadmap for sustained anger management mastery. This strategic approach involves intentional steps, resilience-building, and a commitment to personal growth, ensuring that the journey toward emotional balance becomes an enduring and transformative odyssey.

Reflection and Self-Awareness as Foundations

The foundation of any enduring action plan is rooted in self-awareness and reflection. To craft a plan that spans the long term, parents must engage in ongoing self-reflection. This involves regularly assessing emotional triggers, identifying patterns of response, and gaining insights into the root causes of anger. By cultivating self-awareness, parents lay the groundwork for informed and sustainable action.

Setting Realistic and Achievable Goals

Long-term success in anger management hinges on the establishment of realistic and achievable goals. These goals should be specific, measurable, and tailored to the individual circumstances of each parent. Whether it's a commitment to more effective communication, a reduction in reactive behaviors, or the cultivation of specific coping mechanisms, setting clear goals provides a roadmap for progress.

Continuous Learning and Skill Development

The journey toward lasting anger management mastery involves continuous learning and skill development. Parents should actively seek out resources, workshops, and literature that deepen their understanding of anger, its triggers, and effective coping strategies. Skill development may encompass communication techniques, mindfulness practices, and cognitive-behavioral tools. The commitment to learning ensures that parents are equipped with a diverse array of skills for navigating the complexities of their emotions.

Regular Check-Ins and Progress Assessments

An enduring action plan necessitates regular check-ins and progress assessments. Establishing a routine for self-evaluation allows parents to track their progress, identify areas that require attention, and celebrate achievements. Regular check-ins also provide an opportunity for adaptive adjustments to the action plan, ensuring its relevance and effectiveness over time.

Integration of Mindfulness Practices

Mindfulness practices play a pivotal role in long-term anger management. Cultivating mindfulness involves being fully present in the moment, observing thoughts and emotions without judgment, and responding intentionally. Integrating mindfulness into daily life fosters emotional regulation, resilience, and an increased capacity to navigate challenging situations with composure.

Building a Support System

Sustainable anger management mastery is not a solitary endeavor. Building and maintaining a robust support system is crucial for long-term success. This support system may include family members, friends, mentors, or fellow parents who understand the journey. Regular communication with this support network provides avenues for shared experiences, advice, and encouragement during challenging times.

Embracing Professional Guidance

Long-term success often involves the embrace of professional guidance. Engaging with therapists, counselors, or anger management specialists provides an ongoing source of expert support. Professionals can offer tailored strategies, facilitate deeper insights, and guide parents through the intricacies of their emotional landscapes. Regular sessions ensure that parents receive consistent and personalized guidance throughout their journey.

Creating Rituals and Routines

Incorporating rituals and routines into daily life contributes to the sustainability of an action plan. These rituals may include morning reflections, mindfulness exercises, or designated times for self-care. Creating a structured framework establishes a sense of predictability and control, fostering emotional stability over the long term.

Flexibility and Adaptability

Long-term success in anger management requires flexibility and adaptability. Life is dynamic, and circumstances evolve. Parents should be prepared to adapt their action plans to accommodate changes in family dynamics, personal circumstances, or external stressors. An action plan that can evolve ensures its continued relevance and effectiveness.

Teaching and Modeling for Children

An enduring action plan extends beyond personal benefits—it becomes a legacy that parents impart to their children. Modeling healthy anger management strategies and openly discussing emotions with children contributes to a positive family culture. By teaching children how to navigate their emotions effectively, parents create a generational impact that transcends the immediate family context.

Regular Review and Evolution of the Plan

An action plan is not static; it should evolve in tandem with personal growth and changing circumstances. Regularly reviewing the plan and making necessary adjustments ensure its alignment with current goals and objectives. This iterative process reflects a commitment to continuous improvement and long-term emotional mastery.

Celebrating Milestones and Acknowledging Challenges

Long-term success is marked by both milestones and challenges. Celebrating achievements, no matter how small, reinforces positive behavior and motivates continued effort. Simultaneously, acknowledging challenges with self-compassion and resilience fosters a mindset that views setbacks as opportunities for growth rather than insurmountable obstacles.

In the expansive landscape of anger management, creating a long-term action plan is akin to planting seeds of enduring change. Through self-awareness, continuous learning, and the cultivation of a robust support system, parents ensure that the journey toward emotional mastery is not a destination but a lifelong commitment. In the intentional steps of crafting and revising a comprehensive action plan, parents find the power to transform conflicts into opportunities for growth, anger into constructive change, and the ongoing journey of parenting into a symphony of harmonious relationships that unfolds across the ebbs and flows of family life.

8.1.1 Setting Realistic Goals

Embarking on the journey of anger management demands not only courage but a strategic approach grounded in realistic and achievable goals. In this chapter, we delve into the intricacies of setting realistic goals, recognizing that the path to emotional mastery for parents is a nuanced expedition requiring intentional planning, self-awareness, and a commitment to sustained personal growth.

Understanding the Essence of Realistic Goals

Realistic goals form the cornerstone of effective anger management. While the aspiration to eliminate anger entirely may seem commendable, it is often impractical. Realistic goals acknowledge the inherent human experience of emotions, emphasizing the development of healthier responses to anger rather than its complete eradication. These goals set the stage for sustainable change, fostering resilience and personal growth.

Cultivating Self-Awareness as a Prerequisite

Before setting goals, parents must embark on a journey of self-discovery and self-awareness. Understanding the triggers, patterns, and root causes of anger is crucial. Through reflection and introspection, parents gain insights into their emotional landscape, laying the foundation for setting goals that align with their unique circumstances and aspirations.

The Specificity and Clarity of Goals

Realistic goals are specific and clear, providing a roadmap for tangible progress. Rather than vague aspirations like "be less angry," parents should define precise objectives. For example, a specific goal could be "respond to conflicts with active listening and assertiveness rather than reactive anger." Clarity in goals ensures that parents can measure their progress and celebrate achievements along the way.

Measurable Benchmarks for Progress Tracking

The journey toward emotional mastery involves measurable benchmarks. Establishing quantifiable criteria allows parents to track their progress objectively. Measurable goals might include monitoring the frequency and intensity of anger episodes, assessing the effectiveness of implemented strategies, or gauging improvements in communication with family members. These benchmarks provide a quantifiable lens through which parents can gauge the efficacy of their anger management efforts.

Tailoring Goals to Individual Circumstances

Realistic goals are inherently personal and tailored to individual circumstances. Acknowledging that every parent's journey is unique, goals should reflect the specific challenges, triggers, and strengths of the individual. Tailoring goals to individual circumstances ensures relevance and fosters a sense of ownership, as parents are more likely to commit to goals that resonate with their personal experiences.

Balancing Ambition with Achievability

Setting realistic goals involves striking a delicate balance between ambition and achievability. While it's essential to challenge oneself, overly ambitious goals can lead to frustration and disillusionment. Parents should identify objectives that push them beyond their comfort zones but remain within the realm of attainability. This balance cultivates a sense of empowerment, as parents experience the satisfaction of achieving milestones on their journey.

Prioritizing and Sequencing Goals

Realistic goal-setting requires prioritization and sequencing. Parents should identify which aspects of anger management are most pressing or impactful in their lives and focus on those initially. Prioritizing goals ensures that efforts are concentrated where they can make the most significant difference. Sequencing goals allows for a gradual and sustainable progression toward emotional mastery.

Incorporating Short-Term and Long-Term Goals

An effective strategy involves integrating both short-term and long-term goals. Short-term goals provide immediate objectives that contribute to the overall journey, offering quick wins and building momentum. Long-term goals, on the other hand, set the trajectory for sustained progress over an extended period. The synergy between short-term and long-term goals ensures a dynamic and balanced approach to anger management.

Flexibility and Adaptability in Goal Adjustment

The path to emotional mastery is dynamic, requiring flexibility and adaptability. Realistic goals embrace the idea that circumstances, triggers, and priorities may evolve. Parents should be prepared to adjust their goals as needed, recognizing that adaptability is a strength, not a weakness. This fluidity ensures that the goals remain relevant and responsive to the ever-changing landscape of family life.

Celebrating Achievements and Practicing Self-Compassion

Realistic goal-setting involves celebrating achievements along the way. Recognizing and acknowledging progress reinforces positive behavior and motivates continued effort. Equally important is practicing self-compassion during moments of setback. Realistic goals understand that setbacks are inevitable and view them as opportunities for learning and growth rather than reasons for discouragement.

Incorporating Goal-Setting into Daily Practices

Effective anger management involves the integration of goal-setting into daily practices. Whether through morning reflections, journaling, or regular check-ins, incorporating goal-setting into daily routines reinforces commitment and mindfulness. Daily practices create a structured framework that aligns with the objectives of emotional mastery.

Seeking Professional Guidance in Goal Refinement

Setting realistic goals often benefits from professional guidance. Therapists, counselors, or anger management specialists can provide insights, expertise, and support in refining and adjusting goals. Professional guidance ensures that goals are rooted in evidence-based practices and tailored to the specific needs of each individual.

In the empowering journey of anger management, setting realistic goals acts as a guiding compass, steering parents toward emotional mastery with intention and purpose. Through self-awareness, specificity, measurable benchmarks, and adaptability, parents create a roadmap that transcends the immediate challenges, fostering lasting change and personal growth. In the intentional steps of realistic goal-setting, parents find the power to transform conflicts into opportunities for growth, anger into constructive change, and the ongoing journey of parenting into a symphony of harmonious relationships.

8.1.2 Tracking Progress

Celebrating Progress in Anger Management for Parents

Embarking on the path of anger management is a profound journey that demands not only introspection but also a commitment to transformation. In this chapter, we explore the intricate process of tracking progress—a navigational tool that allows parents to assess, celebrate, and refine their efforts in the ongoing quest to be the masters of their emotions.

The Importance of Tracking Progress

Tracking progress in anger management is akin to having a compass in an unfamiliar terrain—it provides direction, reveals patterns, and celebrates the milestones achieved. By diligently monitoring one's emotional landscape, parents gain valuable insights into the effectiveness of their strategies, identify areas for improvement, and cultivate a heightened self-awareness that forms the bedrock of lasting change.

Establishing a Tracking System

The first step in tracking progress is to establish a systematic approach. This involves creating a tracking system that aligns with individual goals and preferences. Whether through journaling, digital apps, or daily reflections, a structured system allows parents to document emotional experiences, responses to triggers, and the implementation of coping strategies. Consistency in tracking creates a comprehensive record of the anger management journey.

Quantifiable Metrics for Objective Assessment

To enhance the effectiveness of progress tracking, incorporating quantifiable metrics provides an objective basis for assessment. Metrics may include the frequency and intensity of anger episodes, the duration of emotional recovery, or the successful application of specific coping mechanisms. By quantifying aspects of the anger management journey, parents can tangibly measure their progress and identify patterns over time.

Reflective Journaling for Insightful Exploration

Journaling serves as a powerful tool for tracking progress with a qualitative lens. Encouraging parents to engage in reflective journaling allows for a deeper exploration of emotions, triggers, and the effectiveness of coping strategies. Describing the context of anger episodes, emotional responses, and reflections on the outcomes provides a rich source of data for self-analysis and growth.

Regular Check-Ins

Incorporating regular check-ins into the routine is a habit of self-reflection that fortifies progress tracking. Scheduled moments of introspection, whether daily, weekly, or monthly, offer opportunities for parents to review their tracking records, assess trends, and celebrate achievements. Regular check-ins transform progress tracking from a task into a dynamic and evolving practice.

Measuring Changes in Reactive Patterns

One of the primary objectives of progress tracking is to measure changes in reactive patterns. By examining how responses to triggers evolve over time, parents can identify shifts in behavior, emotional regulation, and communication. Recognizing even subtle changes in reactive patterns is a testament to the transformative power of intentional anger management efforts.

Celebrating Achievements

Celebrating achievements, both big milestones and small wins, is a pivotal aspect of progress tracking. Acknowledging successful implementations of coping strategies, instances of effective communication, or periods of emotional balance reinforces positive behavior. These celebrations serve as motivational markers, encouraging parents to persist in their journey.

Learning from Setbacks

Equally important in progress tracking is learning from setbacks. The journey toward emotional mastery is not linear, and setbacks offer valuable opportunities for growth. Examining instances of heightened anger, understanding the triggers, and identifying alternative responses contribute to an evolving and adaptive approach to anger management.

Adaptability and Flexibility in the Tracking Process

The process of tracking progress should embody adaptability and flexibility. As circumstances change, goals evolve, and new insights emerge, the tracking system should be flexible enough to accommodate these shifts. An adaptive approach ensures that the tracking process remains relevant and supportive of the dynamic nature of personal growth.

Feedback Loops

Incorporating feedback loops into progress tracking involves seeking input from support systems. Family members, friends, or mentors can provide valuable perspectives on observed changes in behavior and emotional regulation. These external viewpoints offer a holistic understanding of progress and may highlight areas for further exploration and improvement.

Professional Guidance

For a comprehensive view of progress, seeking professional guidance is beneficial. Therapists, counselors, or anger management specialists can provide expert insights, validate achievements, and offer guidance in refining strategies. Professional support ensures that the tracking process aligns with evidence-based practices and contributes to the overall success of anger management efforts.

Cultivating a Growth Mindset

Progress tracking, at its core, is about cultivating a growth mindset—a belief in the capacity for change and continuous improvement. Embracing the journey with openness and resilience positions setbacks as stepping stones and achievements as markers of personal evolution. A growth mindset fosters a positive and forward-looking perspective, vital for sustained progress.

In the seas of emotional mastery, tracking progress serves as the compass that guides parents through the ebbs and flows of their anger management journey. Through systematic tracking, objective assessment, and a commitment to reflection, parents gain insights, celebrate achievements, and refine their approach to anger. In the intentional steps of tracking progress, parents find the power to transform conflicts into opportunities for growth, anger into constructive change, and the ongoing journey of parenting into a symphony of harmonious relationships that unfolds with each navigated wave of emotional evolution.

8.2 Preventing Relapses

The journey toward mastering one's emotions, especially in the context of parenting, is a voyage marked by progress, setbacks, and the potential for relapses. In this chapter, we delve into the intricacies of preventing relapses in anger management, exploring strategies and insights that empower parents to navigate the seas of emotional regulation with resilience and foresight.

Understanding the Dynamics of Relapse

To prevent relapses effectively, it's essential to understand the dynamics at play. Relapses in anger management often occur when individuals revert to old patterns of behavior in response to triggers or stressors. These patterns are deeply ingrained and can resurface during moments of heightened emotion. Acknowledging the potential for relapse is the first step in building a proactive strategy to prevent it.

Ongoing Self-Reflection

The cornerstone of preventing relapses lies in ongoing self-reflection—a continuous examination of emotional triggers, responses, and the efficacy of coping strategies. Regular self-reflection serves as a sentinel of awareness, allowing parents to identify early warning signs and make preemptive adjustments to their anger management approach. By staying attuned to their emotional landscape, parents can intercept potential relapses before they gain momentum.

Identifying Triggers and Vulnerabilities

Understanding specific triggers and vulnerabilities is paramount in preventing relapses. Triggers can be external, such as stressful situations or conflicts, or internal, stemming from personal insecurities or unmet needs. Identifying these triggers enables parents to implement targeted strategies and develop coping mechanisms tailored to the unique challenges they may face. Recognizing vulnerabilities allows for a proactive stance in addressing potential relapse triggers.

Creating a Crisis Prevention Plan

Anticipating potential crisis points and creating a crisis prevention plan is a proactive strategy to thwart relapses. This plan may involve predetermined steps to take during moments of escalating anger, such as stepping away from the situation, engaging in deep breathing exercises, or seeking support from a trusted individual. A crisis prevention plan provides a structured response mechanism, helping parents regain control in challenging moments.

Building a Support Network

A robust support network acts as a bulwark against relapses. Engaging with family members, friends, or mentors who understand the journey of anger management provides a valuable support system. These allies can offer perspectives, encouragement, and assistance in implementing preventive strategies. The collective strength of a support network enhances resilience and reduces the likelihood of succumbing to relapses.

Mindful Practices

Incorporating mindfulness practices into daily life is a powerful tool for preventing relapses. Mindfulness involves anchoring oneself in the present moment, observing thoughts and emotions without judgment. Mindful practices, such as meditation or mindful breathing, enhance emotional regulation and create a buffer against impulsive reactions. By cultivating mindfulness, parents build a mental resilience that serves as a protective shield against relapses.

Stress Management Techniques

Stress is a common precursor to anger, and effective stress management techniques play a pivotal role in preventing relapses. These techniques may include regular physical exercise, engaging in hobbies, or practicing relaxation exercises. By proactively managing stress, parents reduce the likelihood of reaching a boiling point and, consequently, mitigate the risk of relapses in anger management.

Learning from Setbacks

Setbacks are an inevitable part of any transformative journey, and preventing relapses involves learning from these moments of challenge. Instead of viewing setbacks as failures, parents can embrace them as opportunities for growth. Analyzing the circumstances surrounding a relapse, identifying triggers, and adjusting strategies contribute to a resilient and adaptive approach to anger management.

Adapting and Refining Strategies

An evolutionary approach to anger management involves a continuous adaptation and refinement of strategies. What worked in the past may need adjustment as circumstances change or new insights emerge. The ability to adapt and refine strategies in response to evolving challenges is a key element in preventing relapses and ensuring the ongoing efficacy of anger management efforts.

Regular Check-Ins and Progress Assessments

Regular check-ins and progress assessments serve as the compass of prevention. These intentional moments of self-evaluation provide opportunities to review the effectiveness of preventive strategies, celebrate successes, and identify areas for improvement. By staying vigilant and proactive, parents maintain a vigilant stance against relapses, steering the course of their anger management journey with foresight and resilience.

Seeking Professional Guidance in Times of Vulnerability

During times of heightened vulnerability, seeking professional guidance becomes a valuable resource. Therapists, counselors, or anger management specialists can offer targeted strategies, insights, and support to navigate particularly challenging periods. Professional guidance provides an additional layer of assistance during moments of increased risk of relapse.

Cultivating a Resilient Mindset

A resilient mindset is foundational to preventing relapses. Cultivating resilience involves viewing challenges as opportunities for growth, embracing setbacks as temporary, and maintaining a positive outlook on the overall journey. A resilient mindset positions parents to weather emotional storms with fortitude, reducing the impact and duration of potential relapses.

In the seas of emotional mastery, preventing relapses is akin to navigating with a skilled hand, a vigilant eye, and a compass calibrated with self-awareness. Through ongoing self-reflection, crisis prevention plans, mindfulness practices, and the support of allies, parents can create a resilient vessel that withstands the waves of triggers and stressors. In the intentional steps of preventing relapses, parents find the power to transform conflicts into opportunities for growth, anger into constructive change, and the ongoing journey of parenting into a symphony of harmonious relationships that sails smoothly through the ebbs and flows of family life.

8.2.1 Identifying Potential Challenges

Embarking on the journey of anger management requires not only courage but a keen awareness of the potential challenges that may arise along the way. In this chapter, we explore the intricate landscape of identifying potential challenges in the realm of anger management for parents—a roadmap that empowers individuals to navigate the complexities with foresight, resilience, and a commitment to lasting emotional mastery.

Anticipating the Complexity of Parenting Dynamics

Parenting, by its nature, is a complex and demanding role that presents a myriad of challenges. Anticipating the dynamics of parenting is crucial in understanding the potential triggers and stressors that may contribute to anger. The multifaceted responsibilities, coupled with the diverse needs of children, create a fertile ground for emotional reactions. Identifying the complexity of parenting dynamics allows parents to proactively address challenges that may arise.

Recognizing Individual Triggers and Vulnerabilities

Each parent carries a unique set of triggers and vulnerabilities, stemming from personal experiences, insecurities, or unresolved issues. Identifying these individual triggers is a critical step in preventing potential challenges. Whether it's stress from work, financial concerns, or unresolved emotions from the past, recognizing and addressing individual triggers provides a tailored approach to anger management.

Understanding the Impact of External Stressors

External stressors, such as financial difficulties, health issues, or external conflicts, can significantly impact a parent's emotional well-being. Understanding the potential impact of these stressors is essential in preparing for potential challenges in anger management. By recognizing the connection between external stressors and emotional reactions, parents can develop strategies to mitigate the effects and maintain emotional balance.

Navigating Relationship Dynamics within the Family

Family dynamics play a pivotal role in the anger management journey. Interactions with a partner, children, or extended family members can become potential sources of stress and conflict. Identifying potential challenges within relationship dynamics involves recognizing communication patterns, setting boundaries, and fostering open dialogue. Navigating these dynamics with awareness enables parents to address challenges proactively and maintain harmonious relationships.

Balancing Work-Life Responsibilities

The delicate balance between work and family life is a common challenge for many parents. Juggling professional responsibilities with parenting duties can lead to exhaustion and heightened stress levels. Identifying the challenges associated with work-life balance allows parents to implement strategies for self-care, time management, and effective communication to prevent the spillover of stress into family interactions.

Managing Time Pressures and Demands

Time pressures and demanding schedules can contribute to heightened emotions and potential anger triggers. Identifying the challenges associated with time management involves assessing priorities, setting realistic expectations, and establishing boundaries. Recognizing the limitations of time allows parents to make intentional choices, reducing the likelihood of feeling overwhelmed and reactive.

Addressing Unmet Needs and Self-Care Deficits

Parents, often immersed in the care of others, may neglect their own needs and well-being. Identifying challenges related to unmet needs and self-care deficits is crucial. Recognizing signs of burnout, fatigue, or emotional exhaustion allows parents to prioritize self-care practices, fostering resilience and preventing potential challenges in anger management.

Cultural and Societal Influences on Parenting Styles

Cultural and societal influences play a significant role in shaping parenting styles and expectations. Identifying potential challenges arising from cultural or societal pressures allows parents to navigate these influences consciously. Understanding the impact of cultural norms, societal expectations, and external judgments empowers parents to align their parenting approach with their values while mitigating external sources of stress.

Recognizing the Influence of Past Traumas

Past traumas, whether unresolved or unacknowledged, can manifest as potential challenges in anger management. Recognizing the influence of past traumas involves exploring one's own history and seeking support when needed. Addressing past wounds allows parents to approach their current roles with emotional resilience and a proactive stance in managing potential triggers.

Effectively Communicating with Co-Parents or Ex-Partners

For parents who share custody or have co-parenting arrangements, effective communication is essential. Identifying potential challenges in communication with co-parents or ex-partners involves recognizing communication styles, setting clear boundaries, and fostering a collaborative approach. Proactive communication strategies prevent misunderstandings and reduce the likelihood of conflicts that may trigger anger.

The Influence of Technology on Family Interactions

In the digital age, the influence of technology on family interactions is a growing challenge. Screen time, social media, and constant connectivity can impact the quality of family relationships. Identifying potential challenges related to technology use allows parents to establish healthy boundaries, promote face-to-face interactions, and create a balanced family environment.

Addressing Resistance to Change and New Strategies

Implementing new strategies and embracing change can be met with resistance, both internally and externally. Identifying potential challenges related to resistance allows parents to navigate this aspect of the journey with patience and persistence. Acknowledging the discomfort associated with change and addressing resistance fosters a more adaptive and proactive approach to anger management.

The Role of Mental Health Challenges

Mental health challenges, such as anxiety or depression, can exacerbate emotional reactions and contribute to potential challenges in anger management. Recognizing the role of mental health in anger dynamics involves seeking professional support, practicing self-awareness, and implementing coping strategies tailored to individual mental health needs.

In the expansive landscape of anger management for parents, identifying potential challenges is akin to charting a course through diverse terrains with awareness and foresight. By recognizing the intricacies of parenting dynamics, individual triggers, external stressors, and the multifaceted aspects of family life, parents empower themselves to navigate the journey with intention. In the intentional steps of identifying potential challenges, parents find the power to transform conflicts into opportunities for growth, anger into constructive change, and the ongoing journey of parenting into a symphony of harmonious relationships.

8.2.2 Staying Committed to Personal Growth

The journey of anger management is not a destination but a continuous path of self-discovery, resilience, and personal growth. In this chapter, we delve into the art of staying committed to personal growth—a perennial garden that blooms with intention, nurturance, and an unwavering dedication to mastering emotions for parents.

Embracing Anger as a Catalyst for Growth

To stay committed to personal growth in anger management, it's essential to reframe anger as a catalyst for growth rather than a hindrance. Anger, when approached with awareness, becomes a signal pointing towards unmet needs, unresolved issues, or areas for improvement. Embracing anger as a teacher invites parents to explore its roots, fostering a mindset that views challenges as stepping stones for personal evolution.

Setting Realistic Expectations for the Journey

The commitment to personal growth requires setting realistic expectations for the journey. Acknowledging that transformation is a gradual process helps manage frustrations and prevents feelings of inadequacy. Setting achievable goals and milestones allows parents to celebrate incremental successes, reinforcing the commitment to continuous improvement.

Cultivating a Growth Mindset

A growth mindset is foundational to staying committed to personal growth. Viewing challenges as opportunities for learning and growth reframes setbacks as valuable experiences. Rather than perceiving difficulties as roadblocks, a growth mindset encourages parents to extract lessons from every situation, fostering resilience and an unwavering dedication to self-improvement.

Prioritizing Self-Reflection as a Daily Practice

The commitment to personal growth is sustained through the daily practice of self-reflection. Creating dedicated moments for introspection allows parents to assess their emotional landscape, identify triggers, and reflect on the effectiveness of implemented strategies. Regular self-reflection serves as a compass, guiding the course of personal growth with intention and mindfulness.

Celebrating Small Wins Along the Journey

Personal growth is often marked by small wins that accumulate over time. Celebrating these victories, no matter how modest, reinforces the commitment to the journey. Whether it's successfully navigating a challenging situation or implementing a new coping strategy, acknowledging and celebrating small wins cultivates a positive momentum that propels parents forward on the path of self-mastery.

Creating a Supportive Network for Encouragement

Staying committed to personal growth is fortified by a supportive network. Surrounding oneself with individuals who understand the journey, offer encouragement, and share insights creates a nurturing environment. A supportive network provides validation, motivation, and a sense of belonging, all of which contribute to the unwavering commitment to personal growth.

Incorporating Growth into Daily Practices

The commitment to personal growth is woven into the fabric of daily practices. Integrating growth-oriented activities, such as mindfulness exercises, journaling, or self-care routines, reinforces the dedication to self-improvement. Daily practices become rituals that anchor the commitment to personal growth in the midst of life's busyness.

Accepting Imperfection as a Stepping Stone

Personal growth is a journey marked by imperfections and moments of vulnerability. Accepting imperfection as a natural part of the process is integral to staying committed. Rather than viewing imperfections as failures, they become stepping stones for growth. Embracing vulnerability fosters authenticity and resilience, reinforcing the commitment to personal evolution.

Learning from Setbacks as Lessons, Not Failures

Setbacks are inevitable on the path of personal growth. To stay committed, it's crucial to approach setbacks as lessons rather than failures. Each setback offers an opportunity for self-reflection, adjustment, and refinement of strategies. Learning from setbacks transforms challenges into valuable insights, contributing to a more robust and adaptive approach to anger management.

Seeking Professional Guidance for Continued Support

The commitment to personal growth may benefit from professional guidance. Therapists, counselors, or anger management specialists offer expertise, insights, and tailored strategies for ongoing improvement. Seeking professional support is not a sign of weakness but a proactive step in the commitment to personal growth, providing additional tools and perspectives for the journey.

Adapting Strategies Based on Evolving Needs

Personal growth is an evolving process that requires adaptation. Strategies that were effective in the past may need adjustment as circumstances and needs evolve. Staying committed involves a willingness to reassess and refine strategies, ensuring they remain aligned with the evolving landscape of personal growth and anger management.

Maintaining Consistency Through Life's Challenges

Life is replete with challenges that can test one's commitment to personal growth. Whether facing major life changes, unforeseen stressors, or unexpected setbacks, maintaining consistency in growth practices becomes paramount. Consistency through life's challenges demonstrates a steadfast dedication to the journey, even in the face of adversity.

Fostering a Sense of Purpose and Meaning

The commitment to personal growth gains strength when anchored in a sense of purpose and meaning. Connecting the journey of anger management to broader life goals, values, or the desire to create a harmonious family environment provides a deeper motivation. Fostering a sense of purpose infuses the commitment with resilience and enduring determination.

Staying committed to personal growth in anger management is akin to tending to an ever-blooming garden—one that requires intention, care, and an understanding that growth is a perpetual process. By embracing challenges, cultivating a growth mindset, and integrating daily practices that nourish the journey, parents transform anger into opportunities for self-discovery and lasting transformation. In the intentional steps of staying committed to personal growth, parents find the power to navigate the complexities of emotions, transform conflicts into opportunities for growth, and cultivate a perennial garden of harmonious relationships that flourishes with each season of self-evolution.

Conclusion

As we reach the closing notes of our journey through the landscape of anger management for parents, it's fitting to reflect on the symphony of self-mastery—an orchestration of emotions, growth, and the unwavering commitment to be the master of one's own emotional destiny. The echoes of each chapter, the resonance of insights gained, and the harmonies of intentional transformation have painted a canvas of profound change within the realms of parenting and personal evolution.

In the intricate tapestry of emotions, parents have navigated the ebbs and flows, recognizing anger not as an adversary but as a guide—an emissary that whispers of unmet needs, unresolved wounds, and areas awaiting exploration. The commitment to personal growth has been the compass, steering the course through the complexities of parenting, family dynamics, and the multifaceted landscape of the human experience.

The journey began with a welcome—an invitation to embark on a transformative odyssey toward emotional mastery. Purpose illuminated the path, with the understanding that anger, when harnessed and understood, could be a catalyst for growth. The complexities of parenting dynamics, triggers, and the influence of external stressors were dissected, revealing the intricate threads that weave the fabric of familial relationships.

Understanding explosive anger became a cornerstone—a deep dive into the roots and manifestations of intense emotions. The importance of anger management emerged as a beacon, guiding parents toward a place where emotions could be navigated with grace, transforming conflicts into opportunities for understanding and connection.

The symphony then crescendoed into the effects on children—an exploration of the profound impact parental anger has on the emotional landscape of the next generation. The echoes of behavioral consequences, family dynamics, and the far-reaching implications of long-term effects became poignant reminders of the responsibility inherent in the role of a parent.

Diving into the depths of personal triggers, we uncovered the layers of complexity that contribute to explosive emotions. Reflecting on past incidents, common triggers, and recognizing early warning signs became the compass for navigating the seas of emotional regulation. The exploration extended to childhood influences, examining one's upbringing, and the courageous act of breaking generational patterns—a testament to the transformative power of self-awareness.

Stress, as an ever-present companion in parenting, was dissected, revealing the delicate balance required to navigate its impact. Balancing parenting responsibilities, cultivating self-awareness, and the mindful practices of mindfulness became tools for forging a resilient shield against the storms of daily life.

The journey continued with an exploration of various techniques—deep breathing exercises, visualization, effective communication skills, active listening, and constructive expression of emotions. Each technique became a note in the symphony, contributing to the orchestration of emotional harmony. Journaling emerged as a reflective melody, providing a space for introspection and self-discovery.

As we ventured deeper, the role of mindfulness in anger management became a guiding philosophy—a practice that transcends moments of anger into a state of continuous awareness. Developing healthy coping mechanisms became the craft of the artisan, molding responses to triggers with intention and resilience.

In the pursuit of personal growth, recognizing emotional triggers in real-time became an art—a skill honed through self-reflection, adaptability, and a commitment to evolving strategies. The role of professional help was acknowledged as a beacon in times of darkness—a guiding light offering expert insights and tailored approaches.

Preventing relapses became a vigilant watchman, anticipating potential challenges, and fortifying the commitment to growth. Navigating the terrain of setbacks, embracing imperfections, and learning from failures became the pillars supporting the bridge to lasting change.

The commitment to personal growth, as a perennial garden, thrived through the acknowledgment of imperfections, the celebration of small wins, and the cultivation of a growth mindset. The commitment was nurtured through the support of a network, daily practices infused with intention, and the acceptance of setbacks as lessons.

As we conclude this symphony of self-mastery, let us reflect on the transformation woven into the fabric of these pages. The commitment to personal growth is not a static destination but a continuous journey—an unfolding melody of resilience, understanding, and the profound artistry of being the master of one's emotions. May this symphony resonate in the hearts of parents, echoing through the corridors of family life, and radiating the timeless melody of harmonious relationships. The curtain falls on this chapter, but the symphony of self-mastery echoes eternally—a melody composed by the masterful hands of those who dared to embrace the transformative journey of anger management for parents.

www.ingramcontent.com/pod-product-compliance
Lightning Source LLC
Chambersburg PA
CBHW070917260726
48661CB00003B/743